Table of Contents

Free Gift

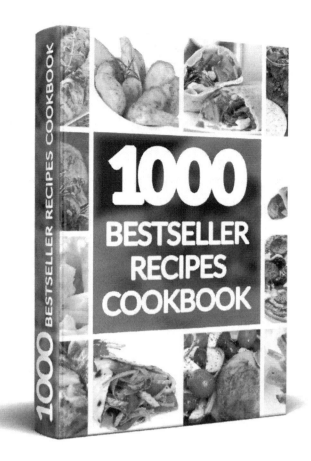

In order to thank you for buying my book I am glad to present you
- 1000 Bestseller Recipes Cookbook -

Please follow this link to get instant access to your Free Cookbook:
http://www.bookbuying.top/

Introduction

Are you looking for a healthy diet that brings you health benefits and improves your appearance at the same time? Do you want to make a change and to transform yourself into a new, healthier and happier person?
Well, if the answer is "yes" to all these questions, you are definitely In the right place!

We searched for the best dietary option and we discover the Ketogenic diet!
This great diet is easy to follow and it will bring you all the benefits you are looking for!

The Ketogenic diet is a low carb one and the best thing about it is that it's very permissive.
If you choose such a diet, you need to know that you can eat a lot of veggies, greens, meat, eggs, nuts, seeds, healthy oils, cheese and berries.
On the other hand, if you opt for a keto diet, you have to stop consuming all kind of grains, sugar, beans, potatoes and other starchy foods.
So, as you can see for yourself, a Ketogenic diet is so easy to follow!

Now that you've made the decision to start a keto life, we recommend you to try something else as well.
We recommend you to cook all your new Ketogenic recipes In the best kitchen pot available on the market these days: In your Crockpot!
Trust us! Your keto meals with taste so great if you make them In your Crockpot!
All your meals with be so delicious, rich, textured and flavored!

So, what do you say?
Are you ready to start your new culinary adventure?
Have fun cooking your keto meals In your Crockpot!

Ketogenic Crockpot Breakfast Recipes

Delicious Breakfast Pie

Preparation time: 10 minutes
Cooking time: 8 hours
Servings: 4

Ingredients:
- 8 eggs, whisked
- 1 yellow onion, chopped
- 1 pound pork sausage, chopped
- 2 teaspoons basil, dried
- 1 tablespoon garlic powder
- A pinch of salt and black pepper
- 1 yellow bell pepper, chopped
- A drizzle of olive oil

Directions:
Grease your Crockpot with the oil, add eggs, onion, pork sausage, basil, garlic powder, salt, pepper and yellow bell pepper, toss, cover and cook on Low for 8 hours. Slice, divide between plates and serve for breakfast.
Enjoy!

Nutrition: calories 251, fat 4, fiber 4, carbs 6, protein 7

Creamy Eggs And Sausage Mix

Preparation time: 10 minutes
Cooking time: 5 hours
Servings: 4

Ingredients:
- 2 garlic cloves, minced
- A pinch of salt and black pepper
- 10 eggs, whisked
- 1 cup cheddar cheese, shredded
- ¾ cup whipping cream
- 12 ounces sausages, sliced
- 1 broccoli head, florets separated and roughly chopped
- A drizzle of olive oil

Directions:
Grease your Crockpot with the oil, add half of the broccoli, sausage and cheese. Add the rest of the broccoli, sausage and cheese. In a bowl, mix the eggs with whipping cream, salt, pepper and garlic, whisk and pour into the pot as well. Cover, cook on Low for 5 hours, divide between plates and serve for breakfast.
Enjoy!

Nutrition: calories 211, fat 7, fiber 4, carbs 5, protein 5

Tasty Spinach Quiche

Preparation time: 10 minutes
Cooking time: 4 hours
Servings: 4

Ingredients:

- 10 ounces spinach
- 2 cups baby Bella mushrooms, chopped
- 1 red bell pepper, chopped
- 1 and ½ cups cheddar cheese, shredded
- 8 eggs
- 1 cup coconut cream
- 2 tablespoons chives, chopped
- A pinch of salt and black pepper
- ½ cup almond flour
- ¼ teaspoons baking soda
- Cooking spray

Directions:

In a bowl, mix the eggs with coconut cream, chives, salt and pepper and whisk. Add almond flour and baking soda and whisk well again. Add cheddar, bell pepper, mushrooms and spinach, toss, transfer to your Crockpot after you've greased it with cooking spray, cover and cook on Low for 4 hours. Slice quiche, divide between plates and serve for breakfast.
Enjoy!

Nutrition: calories 211, fat 6, fiber 6, carbs 6, protein 10

Egg And Bacon Casserole

Preparation time: 10 minutes
Cooking time: 4 hours
Servings: 6

Ingredients:

- 2 cups cheddar cheese, grated
- 1 and ½ cups bacon, cooked and crumbled
- 1 and ½ cups cherry tomatoes, halved
- 1 bunch scallions, chopped
- 1 tablespoon olive oil
- A pinch of salt and black pepper
- 8 eggs
- ½ cup coconut milk

Directions:

In a large bowl, mix the eggs with salt, pepper, milk, scallions, tomatoes, bacon and cheese and whisk well. Add the oil to your Crockpot, add eggs mix, cover and cook on Low for 4 hours. Divide between plates and serve.
Enjoy!

Nutrition: calories 172, fat 5, fiber 4, carbs 6, protein 8

Breakfast Omelet

Preparation time: 10 minutes
Cooking time: 3 hours
Servings: 4

Ingredients:

- Cooking spray
- 6 eggs
- 1 tablespoon coconut milk
- ½ red bell pepper, chopped
- ½ green bell pepper, chopped
- 1 small yellow onion, chopped
- ½ cup ham, chopped
- 1 cup cheddar cheese, shredded
- A pinch of salt and black pepper

Directions:
Grease your Crockpot with cooking spray and spread onion, ham, red and green bell pepper on the bottom. In a bowl, mix the eggs with salt, pepper, cheese and milk, whisk well and pour over veggies and ham. Cover, cook on High for 3 hours, divide between plates and serve for breakfast right away.
Enjoy!

Nutrition: calories 192, fat 6, fiber 5, carbs 6, protein 12

Healthy Veggie Casserole

Preparation time: 10 minutes
Cooking time: 4 hours
Servings: 8

Ingredients:

- 8 eggs
- 4 egg whites
- 2 teaspoons mustard
- ¾ cup almond milk
- A pinch of salt and black pepper
- 2 red bell peppers, chopped
-
- 1 yellow onion, chopped
- 1 teaspoon sweet paprika
- 4 bacon strips, chopped
- 6 ounces cheddar cheese, shredded
- Cooking spray

Directions:
In a bowl, mix the eggs with egg whites, mustard, milk, salt, pepper and sweet paprika and whisk well. Grease your Crockpot with cooking spray and spread bell peppers, bacon and onion on the bottom. Add mixed eggs, sprinkle cheddar all over, cover and cook on Low for 4 hours. Divide between plates and serve for breakfast.
Enjoy!

Nutrition: calories 172, fat 6, fiber 3, carbs 6, protein 7

Mediterranean Frittata

Preparation time: 10 minutes
Cooking time: 4 hours
Servings: 4

Ingredients:
- 8 eggs
- A pinch of salt and black pepper
- ½ cup coconut milk
- 1 teaspoon oregano, dried
- 4 cups baby arugula
- 1 and ¼ cup roasted red peppers, chopped
- ½ cup red onion, chopped
- ¾ cup goat cheese, crumbled
- Cooking spray

Directions:
In a bowl, mix the eggs with milk, oregano, salt and pepper and whisk well. Grease your Crockpot with cooking spray and spread roasted peppers, onion and arugula on the bottom. Add eggs mix, sprinkle goat cheese all over, cover and cook on Low for 4 hours. Divide frittata between plates and serve for breakfast.
Enjoy!

Nutrition: calories 199, fat 3, fiber 6, carbs 6, protein 4

Delicious Egg Scramble

Preparation time: 10 minutes
Cooking time: 6 hours
Servings: 6

Ingredients:
- 12 eggs
- 14 ounces sausages, sliced
- 1 cup coconut milk
- 16 ounces cheddar cheese, shredded
- A pinch of salt and black pepper
- 1 teaspoon basil, dried
- 1 teaspoon oregano, dried
- Cooking spray

Directions:
Grease your Crockpot with cooking spray and spread sausages on the bottom. Crack eggs, add milk, basil, oregano, salt and pepper, whisk a bit, sprinkle cheddar all over, cover and cook on Low for 6 hours. Divide egg scramble between plates and serve.
Enjoy!

Nutrition: calories 177, fat 4, fiber 5, carbs 6, protein 9

Tasty Asparagus Casserole

Preparation time: 10 minutes
Cooking time: 6 hours
Servings: 4

Ingredients:

- 10 ounces cream of celery
- 12 ounces asparagus, chopped
- 2 eggs, hard- boiled, peeled and sliced
- 1 cup cheddar cheese, shredded
- 1 teaspoon olive oil

Directions:
Grease your Crockpot with the oil. Add cream of celery and cheese to the pot and stir. Add asparagus and eggs, cover and cook on Low for 6 hours. Divide between plates and serve for breakfast.
Enjoy!

Nutrition: calories 241, fat 5, fiber 4, carbs 5, protein 12

Tasty Asparagus And Mushroom Casserole

Preparation time: 10 minutes
Cooking time: 5 hours
Servings: 4

Ingredients:

- 2 pounds asparagus spears, cut into medium pieces
- 1 cup mushrooms, sliced
- A drizzle of olive oil
- A pinch of salt and black pepper
- 2 cups coconut milk
- 1 teaspoon Worcestershire sauce
- 5 eggs, whisked

Directions:
Grease your Crockpot with the oil and spread asparagus and mushrooms on the bottom. In a bowl, mix the eggs with milk, salt, pepper and Worcestershire sauce, whisk, pour into the pot, toss everything, cover and cook on Low for 6 hours. Divide between plates and serve right away for breakfast.
Enjoy!

Nutrition: calories 211, fat 4, fiber 4, carbs 6, protein 5

Italian Eggs

Preparation time: 10 minutes
Cooking time: 6 hours
Servings: 4

Ingredients:
- 1 and ½ tablespoon olive oil
- 1 yellow onion, chopped
- 3 garlic cloves, minced
- 27 ounces canned tomatoes, crushed
- 1 tablespoon Worcestershire sauce
- 2 tablespoons tomato paste
- 1 teaspoon basil, dried
- 1 teaspoon oregano, dried
- ¼ teaspoon chili flakes
- A pinch of salt and black pepper
- 4 eggs
- ¼ cup parsley, chopped

Directions:
Heat up a pan with the oil over medium heat, add garlic and onion, stir, cook for 2-3 minutes and transfer everything to your Crockpot. Add tomatoes, tomato paste, Worcestershire sauce, chili flakes, oregano, basil, salt and pepper, cover and cook on Low for 6 hours. Make 4 well In this mix, crack an egg In each, cover and cook on High for 20 minutes more. Sprinkle parsley all over, divide everything between plates and serve for breakfast.
Enjoy!

Nutrition: calories 222, fat 4, fiber 6, carbs 6, protein 10

Incredible Sausage And Bacon Casserole

Preparation time: 10 minutes
Cooking time: 3 hours
Servings: 4

Ingredients:
- 6 bacon slices, chopped
- 6 sausages, sliced
- 3 carrots, chopped
- 2 tablespoons tomato puree
- 1 teaspoon sweet paprika
- 2 leeks, chopped
- 10 ounces canned tomatoes, chopped
- 3 ounces water
- A pinch of salt and black pepper

Directions:
In your Crockpot, mix bacon with sausages, carrots, tomato puree, paprika, leeks, tomatoes, water, salt and pepper, toss, cover and cook on High for 3 hours. Divide between plates and serve for breakfast.
Enjoy!

Nutrition: calories 217, fat 6, fiber 5, carbs 6, protein 16

Spinach And Feta Quiche

Preparation time: 10 minutes
Cooking time: 6 hours
Servings: 8

Ingredients:
- 1 pound chicken, ground
- 10 ounces spinach
- 6 ounces feta cheese, crumbled
- 1/3 cup dill, chopped
- 2 tablespoons onion flakes
- 6 eggs
- 12 ounces coconut milk
- A pinch of salt and black pepper
- Cooking spray

Directions:
Grease your Crockpot with cooking spray. In a bowl, mix chicken with feta, spinach, dill, onion flakes, salt and pepper and stir well. IN a separate bowl, mix the eggs with salt, pepper and milk and whisk well. Add this to chicken mix, toss everything, transfer to your Crockpot, cover and cook on Low for 6 hours. Divide between plates and serve for breakfast.
Enjoy!

Nutrition: calories 251, fat 5, fiber 5, carbs 6, protein 18

Chorizo Casserole

Preparation time: 10 minutes
Cooking time: 4 hours
Servings: 8

Ingredients:
- 1 pound chorizo, chopped
- 1 yellow onion, chopped
- 1 sweet red pepper, chopped
- 2 jalapenos, chopped
- 12 eggs
- 1 cup coconut milk
- ½ cup Mexican cheese, shredded
- A pinch of salt and white pepper
- Cooking spray

Directions:
Heat up a pan over medium- high heat, add chorizo, jalapenos, red pepper and onion, stir, cook for 7 minutes and transfer to your Crockpot after you've greased it with cooking spray. In a bowl, mix the eggs with salt, pepper and milk, whisk well and pour over chorizo mix. Sprinkle cheese, cover pot and cook on Low for 4 hours. Divide between plates and serve hot.
Enjoy!

Nutrition: calories 272, fat 6, fiber 4, carbs 7, protein 22

Spicy Sausage And Eggs Mix

Preparation time: 10 minutes
Cooking time: 5 hours
Servings: 3

Ingredients:
- A drizzle of olive oil
- ¼ pound Mexican spicy sausage, chopped
- ¼ cup green onions, chopped
- A pinch of salt and black pepper
- 6 eggs
- 1 tablespoon cilantro, chopped

Directions:
Heat up a pan with the oil over medium- high heat, add spicy sausage, stir, cook for 6-7 minutes and transfer to your Crockpot. In a bowl, mix the eggs with salt, pepper, green onions and cilantro, whisk well, pour over sausages, cover pot and cook on Low for 5 hours. Divide between plates and serve for breakfast.
Enjoy!

Nutrition: calories 261, fat 6, fiber 6, carbs 8, protein 22

Kale Frittata

Preparation time: 10 minutes
Cooking time: 3 hours
Servings: 4

Ingredients:
- 1 teaspoon olive oil
- 7 ounces roasted red peppers, chopped
- 6 ounces baby kale
- 6 ounces feta cheese, crumbled
- ¼ cup green onions, sliced
- 7 eggs, whisked
- A pinch of salt and black pepper

Directions:
In a bowl, mix the eggs with cheese, kale, red peppers, green onions, salt and pepper, whisk well and pour into the Crockpot after you've greased it with the oil. Cover pot, cook on Low for 3 hours, divide between plates and serve right away.
Enjoy!

Nutrition: calories 261, fat 7, fiber 4, carbs 6, protein 16

Beef Breakfast Bowl

Preparation time: 10 minutes
Cooking time: 4 hours
Servings: 2

Ingredients:
- 4 ounces beef, ground
- 1 yellow onion, chopped
- 8 mushrooms, sliced
- A pinch of salt and black pepper
- 2 eggs, whisked
- 1 tablespoon olive oil
- ½ teaspoon smoked paprika
- 1 avocado, pitted, peeled and chopped
- 12 black olives, pitted and sliced

Directions:
Drizzle the oil In your Crockpot, add onions, mushrooms, beef, salt, pepper and smoked paprika and stir. Add whisked eggs, stir, cover and cook on Low for 4 hours. Divide beef mix into bowls, top each with avocado and black olives and serve for breakfast.
Enjoy!

Nutrition: calories 260, fat 13, fiber 4, carbs 6, protein 43

Salmon Omelet

Preparation time: 10 minutes
Cooking time: 3 hours and 40 minutes
Servings: 3

Ingredients:
- 4 eggs, whisked
- ½ teaspoon olive oil
- A pinch of salt and black pepper
- 4 ounces smoked salmon, chopped

For the sauce:
- 1 cup almond milk
- ½ cup cashews, soaked, drained
- ¼ cup green onions, chopped
- 1 teaspoon garlic powder
- Salt and black pepper to the taste
- 1 tablespoon lemon juice

Directions:
In your blender, mix cashews with milk, garlic powder, lemon juice, green onions, salt and pepper, blend really well and leave aside for now. Drizzle the oil In your Crockpot, add eggs, salt and pepper, whisk, cover and cook on Low for 3 hours. Add salmon, toss a bit, cover, cook on Low for 40 minutes more and divide between plates. Drizzle green onions sauce all over and serve for breakfast.
Enjoy!

Nutrition: calories 200, fat 10, fiber 2, carbs 6, protein 15

Enchilada Pork Breakfast

Preparation time: 10 minutes
Cooking time: 5 hours
Servings: 8

Ingredients:

- ½ cup enchilada sauce
- 1 pound pork, ground
- 1 pound chorizo, chopped
- Salt and black pepper to the taste
- 8 eggs, whisked eggs
- 1 tomato, chopped
- 3 tablespoons olive oil
- ½ cup red onion, chopped
- 1 avocado, pitted, peeled and chopped

Directions:

In a bowl, mix pork with chorizo, stir and spread on the bottom of your Crockpot after you've greased it with the oil. Add enchilada sauce, cover and cook on Low for 3 hours. Add eggs, tomato, onion, salt and pepper, toss well, cover and cook on High for2 hours more. Divide pork and eggs on plates, add avocado on top and serve.
Enjoy!

Nutrition: calories 400, fat 15, fiber 4, carbs 7, protein 25

Beef And Bok Choy Mix

Preparation time: 10 minutes
Cooking time: 5 hours
Servings: 2

Ingredients:

- ½ pounds beef meat, minced
- 2 teaspoons red chili flakes
- 1 tablespoon tamari sauce
- 2 bell peppers, chopped
- 1 teaspoon chili powder
- 2 tablespoons olive oil
- A pinch of salt and black pepper
- 6 bunches bok choy, trimmed and chopped
- 1 teaspoon ginger, grated

Directions:

Heat up a pan with 1 tablespoon oil over medium- high heat, add beef and bell peppers, stir, cook for 10 minutes and transfer to your Crockpot. Add chili flakes, tamari sauce, chili powder, salt, pepper, bok choy, ginger and the rest of the oil, stir, cover and cook on Low for 5 hours. Divide between bowls and serve for breakfast.
Enjoy!

Nutrition: calories 248, fat 14, fiber 4, carbs 7, protein 14

Chorizo And Cauliflower Mix

Preparation time: 10 minutes
Cooking time: 5 hours
Servings: 4

Ingredients:
- 1 pound chorizo, chopped
- 12 ounces canned green chilies, chopped
- 1 yellow onion, chopped
- ½ teaspoon garlic powder
- A pinch of salt and black pepper
- 1 cauliflower head, florets separated and riced
- 4 eggs, whisked
- 2 tablespoons green onions, chopped

Directions:
Heat up a pan over medium heat, add chorizo and onion, stir, brown for a few minutes and transfer to your Crockpot. Add chilies, garlic powder, salt, pepper, cauliflower, eggs and green onions, toss, cover and cook on Low for 5 hours. Divide between bowls and serve for breakfast. Enjoy!

Nutrition: calories 350, fat 12, fiber 4, carbs 6, protein 20

Salami And Eggs Casserole

Preparation time: 10 minutes
Cooking time: 5 hours
Servings: 4

Ingredients:
- 2 tablespoons ghee, melted
- 2 zucchinis, sliced
- Salt and black pepper to the taste
- ½ cup tomatoes, chopped
- 2 garlic cloves, minced
- 1 cup yellow onion, chopped
- ½ teaspoon Italian seasoning
- 3 ounces Italian salami, chopped
- ½ cup kalamata olives, chopped
- 6 eggs, whisked
- 2 tablespoons parsley, chopped

Directions:
Heat up a pan with the ghee over medium heat, add garlic, onions, salt and pepper, stir, cook for a couple of minutes and transfer to your Crockpot. Add salami, tomatoes, zucchini, olives, Italian seasoning and eggs, toss everything a bit, cover and cook on Low for 5 hours. Add parsley, divide between plates and serve.
Enjoy!

Nutrition: calories 333, fat 23, fiber 4, carbs 12, protein 15

Simple Coconut Mix

Preparation time: 5 minutes
Cooking time: 3 hours
Servings: 1

Ingredients:
- 1 teaspoon cinnamon powder
- ½ teaspoon nutmeg, ground
- ½ cup almonds, ground
- 1 teaspoon stevia
- 1 and ½ cup coconut cream
- ¼ teaspoon cardamom, ground
- ¼ teaspoon cloves, ground

Directions:
In your Crockpot, mix coconut cream with cinnamon, nutmeg, almonds, stevia, cardamom and cloves, stir, cover and cook on Low for 3 hours. Divide between bowls and serve.
Enjoy!

Nutrition: calories 200, fat 12, fiber 4, carbs 8, protein 16

Beef And Radish Breakfast

Preparation time: 10 minutes
Cooking time: 3 hours
Servings: 2

Ingredients:
- 1 tablespoon olive oil
- 2 garlic cloves, minced
- ½ cup beef stock
- A pinch of salt and black pepper
- 1 yellow onion, chopped
- 2 cups corned beef, chopped
- 1 pound radishes, cut into quarters

Directions:
Drizzle the oil on the bottom of your Crockpot and add beef. Also add radishes, garlic, stock, onion, salt and pepper, toss, cover and cook on Low for 3 hours. Divide between bowls and serve right away for breakfast.
Enjoy!

Nutrition: calories 240, fat 7, fiber 3, carbs 7, protein 8

Eggs And Brussels Sprouts Breakfast

Preparation time: 10 minutes
Cooking time: 4 hours
Servings: 4

Ingredients:
- 4 eggs, whisked
- Salt and black pepper to the taste
- 1 tablespoon avocado oil
- 2 shallots, minced
- 2 garlic cloves, minced
- 12 ounces Brussels sprouts, sliced
- 2 ounces bacon, chopped

Directions:
Drizzle the oil on the bottom of your Crockpot and spread Brussels sprouts, garlic, bacon and shallots on the bottom. Add whisked eggs, salt and pepper, toss, cover and cook on Low for 4 hours. Divide between plates and serve right away for breakfast.
Enjoy!

Nutrition: calories 240, fat 7, fiber 4, carbs 7, protein 13

Easy Chia Pudding

Preparation time: 10 minutes
Cooking time: 3 hours and 15 minutes
Servings: 2

Ingredients:
- 2 tablespoons coffee
- 2 cups water
- 1/3 cup chia seeds
- 1 tablespoon stevia
- 1 tablespoon vanilla extract
- 2 tablespoons unsweetened chocolate chips
- ¼ cup coconut cream

Directions:
Heat up a small pot with the water over medium heat, bring to a boil, add coffee, simmer for 15 minutes, take off heat and strain Into your Crockpot. Add vanilla extract, coconut cream, stevia, chocolate chips and chia seeds, stir well, cover and cook on Low for 3 hours. Divide between bowls and serve cold for breakfast.
Enjoy!

Nutrition: calories 100, fat 0.4, fiber 4, carbs 3, protein 3

Delicious Chicken Frittata

Preparation time: 10 minutes
Cooking time: 5 hours
Servings: 5

Ingredients:
- 7 eggs
- 3 tablespoons almond flour
- 1 tablespoon olive oil
- A pinch of salt and black pepper
- 2 zucchinis, grated
- ½ cup coconut cream
- 1 teaspoon fennel seeds
- 1 teaspoon oregano, dried
- 1 pound chicken meat, ground

Directions:
In a bowl, mix the eggs with flour, salt, pepper, cream, zucchini, fennel, oregano and meat, whisk well, pour Into your Crockpot after you've greased it with the oil, cover and cook on Low for 5 hours. Slice frittata, divide between plates and serve for breakfast.
Enjoy!

Nutrition: calories 300, fat 23, fiber 3, carbs 4, protein 18

Different Chicken Omelet

Preparation time: 10 minutes
Cooking time: 3 hours
Servings: 2

Ingredients:
- 1 ounce rotisserie chicken, shredded
- 1 teaspoon mustard
- 1 tablespoon homemade mayonnaise
- 1 tomato, chopped
- 2 bacon slices, cooked and crumbled
- 4 eggs
- 1 small avocado, pitted, peeled and chopped
- Salt and black pepper to the taste

Directions:
In a bowl, mix the eggs with salt and pepper and whisk. Add chicken, avocado, tomato, bacon, mayo and mustard, toss, transfer to your Crockpot, cover and cook on Low for 3 hours. Divide between plates and serve.
Enjoy!

Nutrition: calories 270, fat 32, fiber 6, carbs 4, protein 25

Tomatoes Casserole

Preparation time: 10 minutes
Cooking time: 4 hours
Servings: 4

Ingredients:
- 2 teaspoons onion powder
- ¾ cup cashews, soaked for 30 minutes and drained
- 1 teaspoon garlic powder
- ½ teaspoon sage, dried
- Salt and black pepper to the taste
- 1 yellow onion, chopped
- 2 tablespoons parsley, chopped
- 3 garlic cloves, minced
- 1 tablespoon olive oil
- 5 tomatoes, cubed
- ½ teaspoon red pepper flakes

Directions:
In your blender, mix cashews with onion powder, garlic powder, sage, salt and pepper and pulse really well. Add oil to your Crockpot and arrange tomatoes, pepper flakes, garlic, onion, salt, pepper and parsley. Add cashews sauce, toss, cover, cook on High for 4 hours, divide between plates and serve for breakfast.
Enjoy!

Nutrition: calories 218, fat 6, fiber 6, carbs 6, protein 5

Burrito Bowls

Preparation time: 10 minutes
Cooking time: 6 hours
Servings: 6

Ingredients:
- 10 ounces feta cheese, crumbled
- 1 green bell pepper, chopped
- ¼ cup scallions, chopped
- 15 ounces canned tomatoes, chopped
- 1 cup salsa
- ½ cup water
- ¼ teaspoon cumin powder
- ½ teaspoon turmeric powder
- ½ teaspoon smoked paprika
- A pinch of salt and black pepper
- ¼ teaspoon chili powder
- 3 cups spinach leaves, torn

Directions:
In your Crockpot, mix cheese with bell pepper, scallions, tomatoes, salsa, water, cumin, turmeric, paprika, salt, pepper and chili powder, stir, cover and cook on Low for 6 hours. Add spinach, toss well, divide this Into bowls and serve for breakfast.
Enjoy!

Nutrition: calories 211, fat 4, fiber 7, carbs 7, protein 4

Goat Cheese And Mushrooms Casserole

Preparation time: 10 minutes
Cooking time: 4 hours
Servings: 4

Ingredients:
- 1 teaspoon lemon zest, grated
- 10 ounces goat cheese, cubed
- 1 tablespoon lemon juice
- 1 tablespoon apple cider vinegar
- 1 tablespoon olive oil
- 2 garlic cloves, minced
- 10 ounces spinach, torn
- ½ cup yellow onion, chopped
- ½ teaspoon basil, dried
- 8 ounces mushrooms, sliced
- A pinch of salt and black pepper
- ¼ teaspoon red pepper flakes
- Cooking spray

Directions:
Spray your Crockpot with cooking spray and arrange cheese cubes on the bottom. Add lemon zest, lemon juice, vinegar, olive oil, garlic, spinach, onion, basil, mushrooms, salt, pepper and pepper flakes, toss well, cover and cook on Low for 4 hours. Divide between plates and serve for breakfast right away.
Enjoy!

Nutrition: calories 216, fat 6, fiber 5, carbs 7, protein 4

Bell Pepper And Olives Frittata

Preparation time: 10 minutes
Cooking time: 6 hours
Servings: 4

Ingredients:
- 1 pound goat cheese, crumbled
- 2 tablespoons olive oil
- 1 yellow onion, chopped
- ¼ teaspoon turmeric powder
- 3 tablespoons garlic, minced
- 4 eggs, whisked
- 3 red bell peppers, chopped
- A pinch of salt and black pepper
- ½ cup kalamata olives, pitted and halved
- 1 teaspoon basil, dried
- 1 teaspoon oregano, dried
- 1 tablespoon lemon juice

Directions:
Add the oil to your Crockpot, spread cheese all over, add onion, turmeric, garlic, bell pepper, olives, basil, oregano, lemon juice, eggs, salt and pepper, toss a bit, cover and cook on Low for 6 hours. Divide between plates and serve for breakfast.
Enjoy!

Nutrition: calories 271, fat 4, fiber 5, carbs 7, protein 6

Carrot And Zucchini Pudding

Preparation time: 10 minutes
Cooking time: 8 hours
Servings: 4

Ingredients:

- 2 carrots, grated
- 1 and ½ cups almond milk
- 1 zucchini, grated
- A pinch of nutmeg, ground
- A pinch of cloves, ground
- ½ teaspoon cinnamon powder
- 2 tablespoons maple syrup
- ¼ cup walnuts, chopped
- 1 teaspoon vanilla extract

Directions:
In your Crockpot, mix carrots with zucchini, milk, cloves, nutmeg, cinnamon, maple syrup, walnuts and vanilla extract, stir, cover and cook on Low for 8 hours. Divide between bowls and serve for breakfast.
Enjoy!

Nutrition: calories 215, fat 4, fiber 4, carbs 7, protein 7

Pear Breakfast Bowls

Preparation time: 10 minutes
Cooking time: 9 hours
Servings: 2

Ingredients:

- 1 pear, cored and chopped
- ½ teaspoon maple extract
- 2 cups coconut milk
- ½ cup flax meal
- ½ teaspoon vanilla extract
- 1 tablespoon stevia
- ¼ cup walnuts, chopped
- Cooking spray

Directions:
Spray your Crockpot with some cooking spray, add coconut milk, maple extract, flax meal, pear, stevia and vanilla extract, stir, cover and cook on Low for 9 hours. Divide it Into breakfast bowls and serve with chopped walnuts on top.
Enjoy!

Nutrition: calories 150, fat 3, fiber 2, carbs 6, protein 6

Cauliflower Rice Pudding And Salsa

Preparation time: 10 minutes
Cooking time: 2 hours
Servings: 4

Ingredients:
- 1 cup cauliflower, riced
- 1 cup onion, chopped
- 1 cup veggie stock
- 1 red bell pepper, chopped
- 1 green bell pepper, chopped
- 4 ounces canned green chilies, chopped
- A pinch of salt and black pepper

For the salsa:

- 3 tablespoons lime juice
- 1 avocado, pitted, peeled and cubed
- ½ cup cilantro, chopped
- ½ cup green onions, chopped
- ½ cup tomato, chopped
- 1 poblano pepper, chopped
- 2 tablespoons olive oil
- ½ teaspoon cumin, ground

Directions:
In your Crockpot, mix cauliflower with stock and onions, stir, cover and cook on High for 1 hour and 30 minutes. Add chilies, red and green bell peppers, salt and pepper, stir, cover again and cook on High for 30 minutes more. Meanwhile, In a bowl, mix avocado with green onions, tomato, poblano pepper, cilantro, oil, cumin, a pinch of salt, black pepper and lime juice and stir really well. Divide rice mix Into bowls, top each with the salsa and serve.
Enjoy!

Nutrition: calories 140, fat 2, fiber 2, carbs 5, protein 5

Crock Pot Berry Butter

Preparation time: 10 minutes
Cooking time: 5 hours
Servings: 10

Ingredients:
- 5 cups blueberry puree
- 2 teaspoons cinnamon powder
- Zest of1 lemon, grated

- 1 cup coconut sugar
- ½ teaspoon nutmeg powder
- ¼ teaspoon ginger powder

Directions:
Put blueberries In your crock, cover and cook on Low for 4 hours. Add sugar, ginger, nutmeg and lemon zest, stir and cook on High uncovered for 1 hour more. Divide Into jars and serve for breakfast whenever.
Enjoy!

Nutrition: calories 143, fat 2, fiber 3, carbs 3, protein 4

Pumpkin Butter

Preparation time: 10 minutes
Cooking time: 4 hours
Servings: 5

Ingredients:

- 2 teaspoons cinnamon powder
- 4 cups pumpkin puree
- 1 and ¼ cup maple syrup
- ½ teaspoon nutmeg
- 1 teaspoon vanilla extract

Directions:
In your Crockpot, mix pumpkin puree with maple syrup, vanilla extract, cinnamon and nutmeg, stir, cover and cook on High for 4 hours. Divide Into jars and serve for breakfast!
Enjoy!

Nutrition: calories 120, fat 2, fiber 2, carbs 4, protein 2

Cauliflower Rice Pudding

Preparation time: 10 minutes
Cooking time: 3 hours
Servings: 2

Ingredients:

- ½ cup coconut sugar
- 2 cups almond milk
- 1 cup cauliflower rice
- 1 teaspoon vanilla extract
- 1 tablespoons flaxseed meal
- ½ cup raisins
- 1 teaspoon cinnamon powder

Directions:
In your Crockpot, mix almond milk with sugar, cauliflower rice, vanilla, flaxseed meal, raisins and cinnamon, stir, cover and cook on Low for2 hours. Stir your pudding again, cover, cook on Low for 1 more hour, divide between bowls and serve for breakfast.
Enjoy!

Nutrition: calories 160, fat 2, fiber 3, carbs 8, protein 12

Maple And Cauliflower Rice Pudding

Preparation time: 10 minutes
Cooking time: 2 hours
Servings: 2

Ingredients:
- ¼ cup maple syrup
- 3 cups almond milk
- 1 cup cauliflower rice
- 2 tablespoons vanilla extract

Directions:
Put cauliflower rice In your Crockpot, add maple syrup, almond milk and vanilla extract, stir, cover and cook on High for2 hours. Stir your pudding again, divide between bowls and serve for breakfast.
Enjoy!

Nutrition: calories 140, fat 2, fiber 2, carbs 5, protein 5

Fajita Bowls

Preparation time: 10 minutes
Cooking time: 2 hours
Servings: 8

Ingredients:
- 4 ounces canned green chilies, chopped
- 3 tomatoes, chopped
- 1 green bell pepper, chopped
- 1 yellow onion, chopped
- 1 red bell pepper, chopped
- 2 teaspoons cumin, ground
- ½ teaspoon oregano, dried
- 2 teaspoons chili powder
- A pinch of salt and black pepper
- 2 avocados, pitted, peeled and chopped
- Cooking spray

Directions:
Grease your Crockpot with cooking spray, add chilies, tomatoes, bell peppers, onion, cumin, oregano, chili powder, salt and pepper, stir, cover and cook on High for2 hours. Stir again, divide veggies mix Into bowls add avocado on top and serve for breakfast
Enjoy!

Nutrition: calories 140, fat 3, fiber 2, carbs 8, protein 12

Pork Butt And Eggs Mix

Preparation time: 10 minutes
Cooking time: 8 hours
Servings: 4

Ingredients:

- 1 medium pork butt
- 1 teaspoon coriander, ground
- 1 tablespoon oregano, dried
- 1 tablespoon cumin powder
- 2 tablespoons chili powder
- 2 onions, chopped
- A pinch of salt and black pepper
- 1 teaspoon lime juice
- 4 eggs, already fried
- 2 avocados, peeled, pitted and sliced

Directions:
In a bowl, mix pork butt with coriander, oregano, cumin, chili powder, onions and a pinch of black pepper, rub well, transfer to your crock and cook on Low for 8 hours. Shred meat, divide between plates and serve for breakfast with fried eggs and avocado slices on top and with lime juice drizzled at the end
Enjoy!

Nutrition: calories 220, fat 2, fiber 2, carbs 6, protein 2

Leek, Kale and Beef Sausage Breakfast

Preparation time: 10 minutes
Cooking time: 6 hours
Servings: 4

Ingredients:

- 1 and 1/3 cups leek, chopped
- 2 tablespoons olive oil
- 1 cup kale, chopped
- 2 teaspoons garlic, minced
- 8 eggs, whisked
- 1 and ½ cups beef sausage, casings removed and chopped

Directions:
Heat up a pan with the oil over medium- high heat, add leek, garlic and kale, stir, cook for 2 minutes and transfer to your Crockpot. Add eggs and sausage meat, stir everything, cover and cook on Low for 6 hours. Slice, divide between plates and serve for breakfast.
Enjoy!

Nutrition: calories 220, fat 2, fiber 2, carbs 6, protein 10

Crock Pot Meatloaf

Preparation time: 10 minutes
Cooking time: 3 hours
Servings: 4

Ingredients:

- 1 onion, chopped
- 2 pounds pork, minced
- 1 teaspoon red pepper flakes, crushed
- 1 teaspoon olive oil
- 3 garlic cloves, minced
- ¼ cup almond flour
- 1 teaspoon oregano, chopped
- 1 tablespoon sage, minced
- A pinch of salt and black pepper
- 1 tablespoon sweet paprika
- 1 teaspoon marjoram, dried
- 2 eggs

Directions:
Heat up a pan with the oil over medium- high heat, add onion and garlic, stir, cook for 2 minutes and leave aside to cool down. In a bowl, mix pork with salt, pepper, pepper flakes, flour, oregano, sage, paprika, marjoram, eggs, garlic and onion and whisk everything. Shape your meatloaf, transfer to your Crockpot, cover and cook on Low for 3 hours. Leave aside to cool down, slice and serve for breakfast.
Enjoy!

Nutrition: calories 200, fat 3, fiber 2, carbs 7, protein 10

Breakfast Veggies Mix

Preparation time: 10 minutes
Cooking time: 3 hours
Servings: 4

Ingredients:

- 1 and ½ cups red onion, cut into medium chunks
- 1 cup cherry tomatoes, halved
- 2 and ½ cups zucchini, sliced
- 2 cups yellow bell pepper, chopped
- 1 cup mushrooms, sliced
- 2 tablespoons basil, chopped
- 1 tablespoon thyme, chopped
- ½ cup olive oil
- ½ cup balsamic vinegar

Directions:
In your Crockpot, mix onion pieces with tomatoes, zucchini, bell pepper, mushrooms, basil, thyme, oil and vinegar, toss to coat everything, cover and cook on High for 3 hours. Divide between plates and serve for breakfast.
Enjoy!

Nutrition: calories 150, fat 2, fiber 2, carbs 6, protein 5

Butternut Squash Mix

Preparation time: 10 minutes
Cooking time: 8 hours
Servings: 4

Ingredients:
- ½ cup walnuts, soaked for 12hours and drained
- ½ cup almonds
- 1 butternut squash, peeled and cubed
- 1 teaspoon cinnamon powder
- ½ teaspoon nutmeg, ground
- 1 tablespoon coconut sugar
- 1 cup coconut milk

Directions:
In your Crockpot, mix walnuts with almonds, squash, cinnamon, nutmeg, coconut sugar and milk, stir, cover and cook on Low for 8 hours. Divide between bowls and serve for breakfast. Enjoy!

Nutrition: calories 202, fat 3, fiber 7, carbs 14, protein 2

Breakfast Pork And Avocado Mix

Preparation time: 10 minutes
Cooking time: 10 hours
Servings: 4

Ingredients:
- 4 pounds pork butt roast
- 1 tablespoon cumin powder
- 2 tablespoons chili powder
- 1 teaspoon coriander, ground
- 1 tablespoon oregano, dried
- 2 yellow onions, sliced
- 2 avocados, peeled, pitted and sliced

Directions:
In your crock, mix pork butt with chili, cumin, oregano, coriander and onions, toss, cover and cook on Low for 10 hours. Shred meat, divide between plates, top with avocado slices and serve for breakfast.
Enjoy!

Nutrition: calories 270, fat 4, fiber 10, carbs 8, protein 25

Breakfast Pork Salad

Preparation time: 10 minutes
Cooking time: 10 hours
Servings: 4

Ingredients:
- 1 yellow onion, chopped
- 3 pounds pork shoulder
- 1 tablespoon cumin, ground
- 2 tablespoon smoked paprika
- 1 tablespoon chili powder
- 1 tablespoon garlic powder
- 2 teaspoons oregano, dried
- 1 teaspoon allspice, ground
- 1 teaspoon cinnamon powder
- A pinch of salt and black pepper
- Juice of 1 lemon
- 1 romaine lettuce head, leaves torn

Directions:
In your Crockpot, mix pork with onion, cumin, paprika, chili, garlic powder, oregano, allspice, cinnamon, salt, pepper and lemon juice, toss, cover and cook on Low for 10 hours. Shred meat using 2 forks, transfer to a bowl, add lettuce and some of the cooking liquid from the pot, toss, divide between plates and serve on a Sunday for breakfast.
Enjoy!

Nutrition: calories 261, fat 4, fiber 6, carbs 7, protein 29

Carrot And Pineapple Breakfast Mix

Preparation time: 10 minutes
Cooking time: 6 hours
Servings: 10

Ingredients:
- 1 cup raisins
- 6 cups water
- 23 ounces applesauce, unsweetened
- 1/3 cup coconut sugar
- 2 tablespoons cinnamon powder
- 14 ounces carrots, shredded
- 8 ounces canned pineapple, crushed
- 1 tablespoon pumpkin pie spice

Directions:
In your Crockpot, mix carrots with applesauce, raisins, splenda, cinnamon, pineapple and pumpkin pie spice, stir, cover, cook on Low for 6 hours, divide between bowls and serve for breakfast.
Enjoy!

Nutrition: calories 139, fat 2, fiber 3, carbs 8, protein 4

Cauliflower And Mushroom Bowls

Preparation time: 10 minutes
Cooking time: 3 hours
Servings: 6

Ingredients:
- 1 cup cauliflower rice
- 6 green onions, chopped
- 3 tablespoons ghee, melted
- 2 garlic cloves, minced
- ½ pound Portobello mushrooms, sliced
- 2 cups warm water
- A pinch of salt and black pepper

Directions:
In your Crockpot, mix cauliflower rice with green onions, melted ghee, garlic, mushrooms, water, salt and pepper, stir well, cover, cook on Low for 3 hours, divide between bowls and serve for breakfast.
Enjoy!

Nutrition: calories 200, fat 5, fiber 3, carbs 7, protein 4

Sausage, Cranberries And Cauliflower Bowls

Preparation time: 10 minutes
Cooking time:2 hours and 30 minutes
Servings: 12

Ingredients:
- ½ cup avocado oil
- 1 pound pork sausage, ground
- ½ pound mushrooms, sliced
- 6 celery ribs, chopped
- 2 yellow onions, chopped
- 2 garlic cloves, minced
- 1 tablespoon sage, chopped
- 1 cup cranberries, dried
- ½ cup cauliflower florets, chopped
- ½ cup veggie stock

Directions:
Heat up a pan with the oil over medium- high heat, add sausage, stir, brown for a couple of minutes and transfer to your Crockpot. Add mushrooms, celery, onion, garlic, sage, cranberries, cauliflower and stock, stir, cover and cook on High for2 hours and 30 minutes. Divide between bowls and serve for breakfast.
Enjoy!

Nutrition: calories 200, fat 3, fiber 6, carbs 9, protein 4

Ketogenic Crock Pot Main Dish Recipes

Delicious Pork Chili

Preparation time: 10 minutes
Cooking time: 10 hours
Servings: 6

Ingredients:
- 3 garlic cloves, minced
- 2 pounds pork roast
- 2 tablespoons garlic powder
- 3 tablespoons smoked paprika
- ½ cup hot sauce
- 2 tablespoons chili powder
- 2 teaspoons cayenne pepper
- 1 tablespoon cumin, ground
- 1 tablespoon red pepper flakes
- A pinch of salt and black pepper
- 1 red bell pepper, chopped
- 2 yellow onions, chopped
- 1 yellow bell pepper, chopped
- 28 ounces canned tomatoes, chopped
- 14 ounces tomato sauce

Directions:
In your Crockpot, mix pork roast with garlic, hot sauce, paprika, chili powder, garlic powder, cumin, salt, pepper, cayenne, pepper flakes, red and yellow bell pepper, onion, tomatoes and tomato sauce, stir, cover and cook on Low for 10 hours. Shred meat, mix with the rest of the Ingredients one more time, divide between bowls and serve.
Enjoy!

Nutrition: calories 261, fat 7, fiber 4, carbs 8, protein 18

Spiced Pork Ribs

Preparation time: 10 minutes
Cooking time: 8 hours
Servings: 4

Ingredients:
- 4 pounds baby back pork ribs
- 2 teaspoons Chinese five spice powder
- A pinch of salt and black pepper
- ½ teaspoon garlic powder
- 1 jalapeno, roughly chopped
- 2 tablespoons coconut aminos
- 2 tablespoons white vinegar
- 1 tablespoon tomato paste

Directions:
In your Crockpot, mix ribs with salt, pepper, Chinese five spice, garlic powder, aminos, jalapeno, vinegar and tomato paste, toss well, cover and cook on Low for 8 hours. Divide ribs between plates and serve.
Enjoy!

Nutrition: calories 312, fat 7, fiber 7, carbs 8, protein 18

Delicious Pork Stew

Preparation time: 10 minutes
Cooking time: 6 hours
Servings: 4

Ingredients:

- 2 tablespoons coconut oil, melted
- 1 garlic clove, minced
- 1 yellow onion, chopped
- 2 pounds pork loin, cut into medium cubes
- A pinch of salt and black pepper
- 2 tablespoons dried mustard
- 2 tablespoons oregano, dried
- ½ teaspoon nutmeg, ground
- 2 pounds oyster mushrooms
- 2 tablespoons white vinegar
- 1 and ½ cups veggie stock
- ¼ cup coconut milk
- 3 tablespoons capers

Directions:
In your Crockpot, mix oil with garlic, onion, pork cubes, salt, pepper, mustard, oregano, nutmeg, mushrooms, vinegar and stock, stir, cover and cook on Low for 5 hours. Add coconut milk and capers, toss, cover and cook on Low for 1 more hour. Divide between bowls and serve.
Enjoy!

Nutrition: calories 345, fat 7, fiber 5, carbs 14, protein 32

Simple Kalua Pork

Preparation time: 10 minutes
Cooking time: 12hours
Servings: 4

Ingredients:

- 3 pounds pork shoulder
- 1 tablespoon liquid smoke
- 3 tablespoons pink salt

Directions:
In your Crockpot, mix pork shoulder with smoke and salt, rub well, cover and cook on Low for 12hours. Slice pork, divide between plates and serve.
Enjoy!

Nutrition: calories 352, fat 8, fiber 4, carbs 10, protein 27

Tasty Pork Shanks

Preparation time: 10 minutes
Cooking time: 5 hours and 16 minutes
Servings: 4

Ingredients:
- 3 pounds pork shanks
- 1 and ½ tablespoons avocado oil
- 3 cups onion, chopped
- 2 cups carrots, chopped
- 4 garlic cloves, minced
- 1 tablespoon oregano, chopped
- 3 cups mushrooms, sliced
- 2 teaspoons thyme, chopped
- 2 tablespoons basil, chopped
- Zest and juice of 1 lemon
- A pinch of salt and black pepper
- 1 cup pumpkin puree
- 1 cup chicken stock

Directions:
Heat up a pan with ½ tablespoons oil over medium- high heat, add pork shanks, brown them for 8 minutes on each side and transfer them to your Crockpot. Add the rest of the oil, onion, carrots, garlic, oregano, mushrooms, thyme, basil, lemon zest and juice, salt, pepper, pumpkin puree and stock, toss, cover and cook on High for 5 hours. Divide everything between plates and serve. Enjoy!

Nutrition: calories 372, fat 7, fiber 5, carbs 12, protein 37

Simple Bacon And Collard Greens

Preparation time: 10 minutes
Cooking time: 5 hours
Servings: 4

Ingredients:
- ½ tablespoon coconut oil
- 6 bacon slices
- 1 yellow onion, chopped
- 4 garlic cloves, minced
- 2 pounds collard greens, roughly chopped
- 2 cups chicken stock
- 2 tablespoons cider vinegar

Directions:
1. Heat up a pan over medium- high heat, add bacon, cook until it's crispy and transfer to your Crockpot.
2. Heat up the same pan with the oil over medium heat, add garlic and collard greens, toss and cook them for a couple of minutes as well.
3. Add greens to your Crockpot, also add onion, vinegar and stock, toss, cover and cook on Low for 5 hours.
4. Divide between plates and serve.

Enjoy!

Nutrition: calories 273, fat 6, fiber 7, carbs 10, protein 17

Simple Pork And Cauliflower Rice

Preparation time: 10 minutes
Cooking time: 6 hours and 10 minutes
Servings: 4

Ingredients:

- 3 pounds pork roast
- 4 bacon slices, chopped
- A pinch of salt and black pepper
- 6 garlic cloves, minced
- 2 tablespoons liquid smoke

For the cauliflower rice:

- 3 cups cauliflower, riced
- 2 tablespoons chicken stock
- ¼ teaspoon garlic powder
- A pinch of salt

Directions:

In your Crockpot, mix pork with bacon, salt, pepper, garlic and smoke, toss well, cover and cook on High for 6 hours. During the last 10 minutes, heat up a pan over medium heat, add cauliflower, stock, salt and garlic powder, stir, cook for 10 minutes, transfer to your blender and pulse a bit. Slice pork and divide it between plates and serve with cauliflower rice on the side. Enjoy!

Nutrition: calories 362, fat 8, fiber 8, carbs 10, protein 26

Chili Verde

Preparation time: 10 minutes
Cooking time: 8 hours
Servings: 4

Ingredients:

- 2 pounds pork stew meat, chopped
- 3 tablespoons cilantro, chopped
- 2 tablespoons olive oil

- 1 and ½ cups salsa verde
- 5 garlic cloves, minced
- A pinch of salt and black pepper

Directions:

In your Crockpot, mix pork meat with oil, salsa, garlic, salt, pepper and 2 tablespoons cilantro, toss, cover and cook on Low for 8 hours. Add the rest of the cilantro, toss, divide between bowls and serve.
Enjoy!

Nutrition: calories 292, fat 6, fiber 7, carbs 12, protein 22

Tender Pork Loin

Preparation time: 10 minutes
Cooking time: 12hours
Servings: 6

Ingredients:
- 2 yellow onions, cut into wedges
- 5 pounds pork loin
- 1 tablespoon sweet paprika
- 3 cups chicken stock
- A pinch of salt and black pepper

Directions:
In your Crockpot, mix pork loin with onions, paprika, stock, salt and pepper, cover and cook on Low for 12hours. Slice pork, divide it and onions between plates, drizzle cooking juices all over and serve.
Enjoy!

Nutrition: calories 322, fat 6, fiber 6, carbs 9, protein 22

Corned Beef Brisket

Preparation time: 10 minutes
Cooking time: 6 hours and 30 minutes
Servings: 4

Ingredients:
- 2 and ½ pounds beef brisket
- 1 yellow onion, chopped
- 1 celery stalk, roughly chopped
- 1 carrot, sliced
- 1 cup chicken stock
- 1 tablespoon avocado oil
- 1 green cabbage head, cut into medium wedges
- A pinch of salt and black pepper

For the cabbage:

Directions:
In your Crockpot, mix beef with onion, celery, carrot and stock, toss, cover and cook on Low for 6 hours. Meanwhile, spread cabbage wedges on a lined baking sheet, season with salt and pepper, drizzle the oil, toss and bake In the oven at 360 degrees F for 30 minutes. Divide beef brisket between plates, add roasted cabbage on the side and serve.
Enjoy!

Nutrition: calories 251, fat 6, fiber 7, carbs 12, protein 6

Simple Beef Stew

Preparation time: 10 minutes
Cooking time: 4 hours and 30 minutes
Servings: 6

Ingredients:

- 2 pounds beef stew meat, cubed
- 1 teaspoon garlic powder
- A pinch of salt and black pepper
- 1 teaspoon onion powder
- 1 teaspoon thyme, dried
- 2 teaspoons sweet paprika
- 1 yellow onion, sliced
- 8 ounces white mushrooms, sliced
- 1/3 cup coconut cream
- 2 teaspoons red vinegar

Directions:

In your Crockpot, mix beef with garlic powder, salt, pepper, onion powder, thyme and paprika and rub well. Add onion, mushrooms, cream and vinegar, toss a bit, cover and cook on Low for 4 hours and 30 minutes. Divide between bowls and serve.
Enjoy!

Nutrition: calories 322, fat 5, fiber 7, carbs 9, protein 16

Spicy Curry

Preparation time: 10 minutes
Cooking time: 5 hours
Servings: 4

Ingredients:

- 2 and ½ pound beef chuck
- 4 garlic cloves, minced
- 1 red onion, chopped
- 1 Inch ginger piece, grated
- 2 tablespoons curry powder
- 2 cups coconut milk
- 2 tablespoons chili sauce
- A pinch of salt and black pepper

Directions:

In your Crockpot, mix beef chuck with curry powder, chili sauce, salt and pepper and rub well. In your food processor, mix onion with garlic, ginger and coconut milk, pulse well and add over beef mix. Cover pot, cook on Low for 5 hours, stir curry one more time, divide between bowls and serve.
Enjoy!

Nutrition: calories 352, fat 6, fiber 7, carbs 9, protein 18

Beef And Cabbage Stew

Preparation time: 10 minutes
Cooking time: 7 hours
Servings: 5

Ingredients:
- ½ pound bacon, cut into medium strips
- 2 red onions, chopped
- 3 pounds beef chuck roast, cut into medium cubes
- A pinch of salt and black pepper
- 1 garlic clove, crushed
- 1 Savoy cabbage, roughly chopped
- 1 thyme spring
- 1 cup beef stock

Directions:
Arrange bacon on the bottom of your Crockpot. Add onion, garlic, roast pieces, cabbage, thyme, salt, pepper and stock, cover pot and cook on Low for 7 hours. Divide between bowls and serve. Enjoy!

Nutrition: calories 261, fat 7, fiber 6, carbs 8, protein 26

Beef And Veggie Stew

Preparation time: 10 minutes
Cooking time: 6 hours
Servings: 4

Ingredients:
- 1 pound beef meat, cubed
- 1 yellow onion, chopped
- 6 ounces tomato paste
- 2 garlic cloves, minced
- 1 tablespoon thyme, chopped
- 2 carrots, chopped
- 3 celery stalks, chopped
- 2 bay leaves
- 2 tablespoons parsley, chopped
- 2 tablespoons white vinegar
- 1 tablespoon arrowroot powder
- A pinch of salt and black pepper

Directions:
In your Crockpot, mix beef with onion, tomato paste, garlic, thyme, carrots, celery, bay leaves, parsley, vinegar, arrowroot powder, salt and pepper, cover and cook on Low for 6 hours. Divide between bowls and serve.
Enjoy!

Nutrition: calories 300, fat 4, fiber 7, carbs 9, protein 22

Red Curry

Preparation time: 10 minutes
Cooking time: 8 hours
Servings: 4

Ingredients:

- 2 tablespoons coconut oil
- 2 tablespoons red curry paste
- 1 and ½ pounds beef stew meat, cubed
- 3 eggplants, cut into medium chunks
- 10 ounces coconut milk
- 1 teaspoon coconut sugar
- 4 kaffir lime leaves

Directions:
In your Crockpot, mix oil with curry paste, beef stew meat, eggplants, coconut milk, coconut sugar and lime leaves, toss, cover and cook on Low for 8 hours. Divide between bowls and serve. Enjoy!

Nutrition: calories 281, fat 7, fiber 6, carbs 8, protein 22

Tasty Meatballs

Preparation time: 10 minutes
Cooking time: 4 hours
Servings: 4

Ingredients:

- 3 pounds beef, ground
- ¼ cup spinach, chopped
- 1 teaspoon garlic powder
- 2 tablespoons onion, chopped
- A drizzle of olive oil
- A pinch of salt and black pepper
- 20 ounces tomato sauce

Directions:
In a bowl, mix beef with spinach, garlic powder, onion, salt and pepper, stir well and shape medium meatballs. Heat up a pan with the oil over medium- high heat, add meatballs, brown them on all sides, transfer to your Crockpot, cover them with the sauce and cook on Low for 4 hours. Divide meatballs and sauce between plates and serve.
Enjoy!

Nutrition: calories 322, fat 5, fiber 4, carbs 12, protein 22

Simple Shredded Beef

Preparation time : 10 minutes
Cooking time : 5 hours and 10 minutes
Servings: 4

Ingredients:

- 3 and ½ pounds beef roast
- ¼ cup veggie stock
- A pinch of salt and black pepper
- ½ teaspoon cumin, ground
- ½ tablespoon oregano, dried
- ¼ teaspoon ancho chili pepper
- A pinch of cinnamon powder
- ¼ teaspoon smoked paprika
- ½ teaspoon garlic powder
- 2 tablespoon tomato paste
- 1 small yellow onion, chopped
- 1 jalapeno, chopped
- 3 garlic cloves, minced
- ½ cup salsa
- ½ tomato, chopped

Directions:

In your Crockpot, mix beef roast with veggie stock, salt, pepper, cumin, oregano, chili pepper, cinnamon, paprika and garlic powder, toss well, cover and cook on Low for 5 hours. Shred meat, divide between plates and transfer 1 cup of cooking juices to a pan. Heat up cooking juices over medium- high heat, add onion, jalapeno, garlic, salsa and tomato, stir, simmer for 5 minutes and drizzle over shredded meat. Serve right away.
Enjoy!

Nutrition: calories 391, fat 6, fiber 7, carbs 8, protein 27

American Beef Brisket

Preparation time: 10 minutes
Cooking time: 8 hours
Servings: 6

Ingredients:

- 3 pounds beef brisket
- A pinch of salt and black pepper
- 1 teaspoon fennel seeds
- 1 teaspoon cloves
- ½ teaspoon peppercorns
- 1 teaspoon cumin powder
- 1 teaspoon cardamom powder
- 3 tablespoons tomato paste
- ½ teaspoon cinnamon powder
- 1 sweet onion, chopped
- 3 cups beef stock
- ¼ cup coconut vinegar

Directions:

In your Crockpot, mix beef brisket with salt, pepper, fennel, cloves, peppercorns, cumin, cardamom, cinnamon and tomato paste and rub well. Add onion, stock and vinegar, toss, cover and cook on Low for 8 hours. Divide beef brisket and cooking juices between plates and serve.
Enjoy!

Nutrition: calories 392, fat 7, fiber 8, carbs 12, protein 28

Mexican Beef Stew

Preparation time: 10 minutes
Cooking time: 8 hours
Servings: 4

Ingredients:

- 1 pound beef stew meat, cubed
- 3 tomatoes, roughly chopped
- 1 red onion, chopped
- 1 garlic clove, minced
- 5 ounces canned green chilies, chopped
- 2 teaspoons chili powder
- 1 teaspoon cumin powder
- 1 teaspoon oregano, dried
- 2 cups water
- 2 cups beef stock
- A pinch of salt and black pepper

Directions:
Put meat In your Crockpot. Add tomatoes, onion, garlic, chilies, chili powder, cumin powder, oregano, water, stock, salt and pepper, cover and cook on Low for 8 hours. Divide between bowls and serve.
Enjoy!

Nutrition: calories 328, fat 6, fiber 8, carbs 12, protein 28

Indian Beef Mix

Preparation time: 10 minutes
Cooking time: 5 hours
Servings: 4

Ingredients:

- 2 and ½ pounds beef roast
- 2 tablespoons coconut oil, melted
- 2 red onions, chopped
- 1 teaspoon black mustard seeds
- A pinch of salt and black pepper
- 25 curry leaves
- 2 tablespoons lemon juice
- 2 tablespoons garlic, minced
- 1 Inch ginger, grated
- 1 Serrano pepper, chopped
- 1 tablespoon garam masala
- 1 tablespoons coriander powder
- 2 teaspoons chili powder
- 1 teaspoon turmeric powder
- ½ teaspoon black peppercorns, ground
- ¼ cup coconut, unsweetened and shredded

Directions:

In your Crockpot, mix onions with salt, pepper, oil and mustard seeds, stir, cover and cook on High for 1 hour. Add beef roast, curry leaves, lemon juice, garlic, ginger, Serrano pepper, garam masala, coriander, chili powder, turmeric powder and black peppercorns, toss a bit, cover and cook on High for 3 hours more. Add coconut, toss, cover and cook on High for 1 more hour. Divide between bowls and serve.
Enjoy!

Nutrition: calories 300, fat 4, fiber 6, carbs 9, protein 22

Beef Tongue Mix

Preparation time: 10 minutes
Cooking time: 6 hours and 30 minutes
Servings: 4

Ingredients:

- 3 pounds beef tongue, sliced
- 2 jalapeno peppers, chopped
- 1 yellow onion, cut into wedges
- 1 red bell pepper, chopped
- 1 yellow bell pepper, chopped
- 5 garlic cloves, minced
- A pinch of salt and black pepper
- 1 teaspoon Cajun spice
- 7 ounces tomato paste
- 2 cups chicken stock
- 1 tablespoon olive oil
- 1 bunch green onions, chopped

Directions:

In your Crockpot, mix beef tongue with jalapenos, onion, red bell pepper, yellow bell pepper, garlic, salt, pepper, Cajun spice, tomato paste, stock, oil and green onions, toss, cover and cook on High for 6 hours. Divide tongue between plates and serve.
Enjoy!

Nutrition: calories 251, fat 6, fiber 3, carbs 7, protein 4

Ground Beef Soup

Preparation time: 10 minutes
Cooking time: 6 hours
Servings: 4

Ingredients:

- 1 pound beef, ground
- 2 zucchinis, chopped
- 1 carrot, chopped
- 1 yellow onion, chopped
- 1 celery stalk, chopped
- ½ cup veggie stock
- 3 cups water
- A pinch of salt and black pepper
- 29 ounces canned tomatoes, chopped
- 1 tablespoon garlic, minced
- ½ teaspoon oregano, dried
- ½ teaspoon basil, dried

Directions:

Heat up a pan over medium- high heat, add meat, brown on all sides and transfer to your Crockpot. Add water, zucchinis, carrot, onion, celery, stock, salt, pepper, tomatoes, garlic, oregano and basil, stir, cover and cook on Low for 6 hours. Ladle Into bowls and serve.
Enjoy!

Nutrition: calories 271, fat 6, fiber 7, carbs 8, protein 12

Crock Pot Chicken Drumsticks

Preparation time: 10 minutes
Cooking time: 5 hours
Servings: 4

Ingredients:
- 10 drumsticks, skinless
- 1 Inch ginger, grated
- 1 lemongrass stalk, trimmed and roughly chopped
- 5 garlic cloves minced
- 1 cup coconut milk
- 3 tablespoons coconut aminos
- 1 teaspoon five spice
- 1 yellow onion, chopped
- A pinch of salt and black pepper
- ¼ cup scallions, chopped

Directions:
In your Crockpot, mix drumsticks with ginger, lemongrass, garlic, coconut milk, aminos, five spice, onion, scallions, salt and pepper, toss, cover and cook on Low for 5 hours. Divide chicken and sauce between plates and serve right away.
Enjoy!

Nutrition: calories 210, fat 2, fiber 7, carbs 9, protein 16

Special Chicken Soup

Preparation time: 10 minutes
Cooking time: 8 hours
Servings: 10

Ingredients:
- 1 whole chicken, cut into medium pieces
- 20 basil leaves
- 1 lemongrass stalk, roughly chopped
- 4 ginger, slices
- Juice of 1 lime
- A pinch of salt and black pepper
- Water to cover

Directions:
In your Crockpot, mix chicken with basil, lemongrass, ginger, lime juice, salt, pepper and enough water to cover the meat, cover pot and cook on Low for 8 hours. Add more salt, stir, divide between bowls and serve.
Enjoy!

Nutrition: calories 211, fat 5, fiber 4, carbs 7, protein 12

Delicious Slow Cooked Chicken

Preparation time: 10 minutes
Cooking time: 5 hours
Servings: 4

Ingredients:
- 5 chicken drumsticks
- A pinch of salt and black pepper
- 1 teaspoon cayenne pepper
- 4 teaspoons sweet paprika
- 2 teaspoons onion powder
- 2 teaspoons thyme, dried
- 2 teaspoons garlic powder

Directions:
In a bowl, mix cayenne with salt, pepper, paprika, onion powder, thyme and garlic powder and stir. Rub chicken with this spice mix, put them In your Crockpot, cover and cook on Low for 5 hours. Discard bones and serve chicken with a side salad.
Enjoy!

Nutrition: calories 281, fat 4, fiber 6, carbs 7, protein 12

Delicious Bacon Chicken

Preparation time: 10 minutes
Cooking time: 8 hours
Servings: 4

Ingredients:
- 10 bacon slices
- 5 chicken breasts
- 2 tablespoons thyme, dried
- 1 teaspoon oregano, dried
- 1 tablespoon rosemary, dried
- 4 tablespoons olive oil
- A pinch of salt and black pepper

Directions:
In your Crockpot, mix bacon with chicken, thyme, oregano, rosemary, salt ,pepper and half of the oil, toss, cover and cook on Low for 8 hours. Add the rest of the oil, toss, divide chicken and bacon mix between plates and serve.
Enjoy!

Nutrition: calories 271, fat 7, fiber 4, carbs 7, protein 15

Chicken Curry

Preparation time: 10 minutes
Cooking time: 5 hours
Servings: 4

Ingredients:
- 3 pounds chicken thighs, skinless and boneless
- 3 tablespoons green curry paste
- 2 cups coconut milk

Directions:
In your Crockpot, mix chicken thighs with green curry paste and coconut milk, toss well, cover and cook n Low for 5 hours. Divide between bowls and serve right away.
Enjoy!

Nutrition: calories 211, fat 5, fiber 6, carbs 8, protein 12

Yellow Chicken Curry

Preparation time: 10 minutes
Cooking time: 6 hours
Servings: 4

Ingredients:
- 1 and ½ pounds chicken thighs, skinless, boneless and cut into medium chunks
- 1 cup yellow onion, chopped
- 1 cup carrots, chopped
- 1 cup broccoli florets
- 1 cup tomatoes, chopped
- 1 cup red bell pepper, chopped
- 14 ounces coconut milk
- 1 cup tomato sauce
- 1 teaspoon cumin, ground
- 2 teaspoons garlic powder
- 2 teaspoons ginger, grated
- 2 teaspoons coriander, ground
- 1 teaspoon cinnamon powder
- 1 cup water

Directions:
In your Crockpot, mix chicken thighs with onion, carrots, broccoli, tomatoes, red bell pepper, coconut milk, tomato sauce, cumin, garlic powder, ginger, coriander, cinnamon and water, cover and cook on Low for 6 hours. Divide between bowls and serve.
Enjoy!

Nutrition: calories 251, fat 6, fiber 6, carbs 12, protein 26

Delicious Shrimp

Preparation time: 10 minutes
Cooking time: 3 hours and 15 minutes
Servings: 4

Ingredients:

- 1 teaspoon avocado oil
- 1 pound shrimp, shelled
- A pinch of salt and black pepper
- 1 yellow onion, chopped
- 3 garlic cloves, minced
- 1 teaspoon red pepper flakes
- 15 ounces canned roasted tomatoes, chopped
- 1 tablespoon parsley, chopped

Directions:
Heat up a pan with the oil over medium- high heat, add garlic, onion and pepper flakes, stir, cook for 5 minutes and transfer to your Crockpot. Add tomatoes, salt, pepper and parsley to the pot as well, cover and cook on Low for2 hours. Add shrimp, toss, cover and cook on High for 15 minutes. Divide shrimp mix between plates and serve.
Enjoy!

Nutrition: calories 251, fat 4, fiber 6, carbs 8, protein 12

Garlic Shrimp

Preparation time: 10 minutes
Cooking time: 50 minutes
Servings: 4

Ingredients:

- 2 pounds shrimp, peeled and deveined
- 1 tablespoons parsley, chopped
- A pinch of salt and black pepper
- ¼ teaspoon red pepper flakes, crushed
- 1 teaspoon smoked paprika
- 6 garlic cloves, minced
- ¾ cup olive oil

Directions:
In your Crockpot, mix oil, garlic, paprika, salt, pepper and red pepper flakes, stir, cover and cook on High for 30 minutes. Add shrimp and parsley, cover and cook on High for 10 minutes more. Stir again, cover pot again and cook on High for another 10 minutes. Divide between plates and serve.
Enjoy!

Nutrition: calories 200, fat 3, fiber 6, carbs 8, protein 11

Shrimp And Squash Mix

Preparation time: 10 minutes
Cooking time: 2 hours
Servings: 4

Ingredients:

- 2 pound spaghetti squash, peeled, halved and cubed
- 1 yellow onion, chopped
- 1 pound shrimp, deveined and peeled
- 2 and ½ teaspoons lemon- garlic seasoning
- 1 tablespoon olive oil
- 32 ounces chicken stock

Directions:
In your Crockpot, mix stock with lemon garlic seasoning, oil and onion and stir. Add squash, cover and cook on High for 2 hours. Add shrimp, cover and cook on High for 20 minutes. Divide between bowls and serve.
Enjoy!

Nutrition: calories 200, fat 3, fiber 4, carbs 7, protein 11

Simple Oxtail Stew

Preparation time: 10 minutes
Cooking time: 10 hours and 30 minutes
Servings: 4

Ingredients:

- 4 pounds oxtail, cut into medium segments
- 28 ounces canned tomatoes, chopped
- 2 cups water
- 4 teaspoons smoked paprika
- 10 garlic cloves, minced
- 2 tablespoons Italian seasoning
- A pinch of chili powder
- A pinch of salt and black pepper

Directions:
In your Crockpot, mix oxtail with the water, cover and cook on Low for 10 hours. Add garlic, tomatoes, paprika, Italian seasoning, salt, pepper and chili powder, toss, cover and cook on High for 30 minutes more. Divide stew Into bowls and serve.
Enjoy!

Nutrition: calories 261, fat 3, fiber 6, carbs 8, protein 11

Crock Pot Lamb Leg

Preparation time: 10 minutes
Cooking time: 10 hours
Servings: 4

Ingredients:
- 4 pounds lamb leg
- A pinch of salt and black pepper
- 1 and ½ teaspoon thyme, dried
- 2 garlic cloves, minced
- 1 tablespoon olive oil
- 3 cups beef stock
- 3 tablespoons almond flour

Directions:
Put lamb leg In your Crockpot, add salt, pepper, thyme, garlic, oil and stock, stir, cover and cook on Low for 10 hours. Transfer lamb leg to a cutting board, slice and divide between plates. Transfer 2 cups cooking juices to a pot, add almond flour, stir, heat up over medium heat, cook for 1-2 minutes, drizzle over lamb and serve.
Enjoy!

Nutrition: calories 433, fat 12, fiber 4, carbs 6, protein 28

Rabbit Stew

Preparation time: 10 minutes
Cooking time: 6 hours
Servings: 4

Ingredients:
- 1 rabbit, legs removed
- 1 pound spicy sausage, sliced
- 4 carrots, roughly chopped
- 1 yellow onion, chopped
- 2 quarts chicken stock
- ¼ teaspoon red pepper flakes
- 7 ounces mushrooms, sliced
- ¼ teaspoon sweet paprika
- 1 tablespoon coconut oil, melted
- A pinch of salt and black pepper
- A pinch of cayenne

Directions:
Put the oil In your Crockpot and add rabbit. Add sausage, carrots, onion, pepper flakes, stock, mushrooms, paprika, salt, pepper and cayenne, toss, cover and cook on High for 6 hours. Carve rabbit, divide it and veggies Into bowls and serve.
Enjoy!

Nutrition: calories 521, fat 7, fiber 4, carbs 7, protein 38

Bison Roast Soup

Preparation time: 10 minutes
Cooking time: 7 hours
Servings: 4

Ingredients:
- 2 pounds bison roast
- 6 red onions, sliced
- 2 quarts beef stock
- 4 thyme springs
- ½ cup sherry vinegar
- 1 bay leaf
- A pinch of salt and black pepper
- 2 tablespoons olive oil

Directions:
In your Crockpot, mix bison roast with stock, bay leaf and thyme, cover, cook on High for 6 hours, transfer roast to a cutting board, cool it down, shred and transfer to a bowl. Heat up a large pot with the oil over medium- high heat, add onions, stir and cook them for 5 minutes. Add vinegar, stock from the Crockpot, salt, pepper and bison meat, stir and cook for 45 minutes. Divide bison soup Into bowls and serve.
Enjoy!

Nutrition: calories 632, fat 7, fiber 7, carbs 12, protein 37

Easy Lamb Curry

Preparation time: 10 minutes
Cooking time: 6 hours
Servings: 2

Ingredients:
- 3 tablespoons madras curry paste
- 1 yellow onion, sliced
- 10 ounces canned tomatoes, chopped
- 1 tablespoon ginger, grated
- 1 teaspoon cumin seeds
- 1 cinnamon stick
- 1 cup kale, chopped
- 2 lean lamb steaks, chopped

Directions:
In your Crockpot, mix lamb with curry paste, onion, tomatoes, ginger, cumin, cinnamon and kale, toss, cover and cook on Low for 6 hours. Discard cinnamon stick, stir curry, divide between bowls and serve.
Enjoy!

Nutrition: calories 261, fat 4, fiber 4, carbs 8, protein 12

Lamb Shoulder Mix

Preparation time: 10 minutes
Cooking time: 8 hours
Servings: 4

Ingredients:
- 1 and ½ pounds lamb shoulder joint
- 4 carrots, cut into medium chunks
- 10 ounces lamb stock
- A pinch of salt and black pepper
- A handful mint, chopped

Directions:
In your Crockpot, mix lamb with carrots, stock, salt, pepper and mint, cover and cook on Low for 8 hours. Divide lamb and cooking juices between plates and serve.
Enjoy!

Nutrition: calories 281, fat 7, fiber 7, carbs 12, protein 6

Delicious Creamy Chicken

Preparation time: 10 minutes
Cooking time: 6 hours
Servings: 4

Ingredients:
- 1 and ½ pounds chicken thighs, boneless
- 2 teaspoons sweet paprika
- 1 tablespoon chili powder
- 1 teaspoon cumin, ground
- 1 teaspoon coriander, ground
- 1 teaspoon garlic powder
- A pinch of salt and white pepper
- A pinch of cayenne pepper
- 1 cup chicken stock
- 2 red bell peppers, chopped
- ¼ cup lime juice
- ½ cup coconut cream
- 2 tablespoons parsley, chopped

Directions:
In a bowl, mix chicken thighs with paprika, chili powder, cumin, coriander, garlic powder, salt, pepper and cayenne and rub well. Heat up a pan over medium- high heat, add chicken pieces, brown them for a few minutes on each side and transfer to your Crockpot. Add stock, lime juice and top with bell peppers, cover pot and cook on Low for 5 hours and 30 minutes. Add cream and parsley, toss a bit, cover and cook on Low for 30 minutes more. Divide between bowls and serve.
Enjoy!

Nutrition: calories 322, fat 6, fiber 7, carbs 8, protein 18

Creamy Salmon Soup

Preparation time: 10 minutes
Cooking time: 7 hours
Servings: 6

Ingredients:

- 2 tablespoons avocado oil
- 4 leeks, sliced
- 3 garlic cloves, minced
- 6 cups chicken stock
- 2 teaspoons thyme, dried
- 1 pounds salmon, skinless, boneless and cut into medium cubes
- 1 and ¼ cup coconut milk
- A pinch of salt and black pepper

Directions:

Heat up a pan with the oil over medium- high heat, add garlic and leeks, stir, brown for a few minutes and transfer to your Crockpot. Add stock, thyme, salt and pepper, cover and cook on Low for 3 hours. Add coconut milk and salmon, cover and cook on Low for 1 more hour. Ladle Into bowls and serve.
Enjoy!

Nutrition: calories 232, fat 4, fiber 7, carbs 9, protein 11

Crock Pot Shrimp Stew

Preparation time: 10 minutes
Cooking time: 7 hours and 30 minutes
Servings: 6

Ingredients:

- 1 pounds spicy sausage, sliced
- 1 yellow onion, roughly chopped
- 2 celery stalks, chopped
- 2 garlic cloves, minced
- 1 green bell pepper, chopped
- 28 ounces canned tomatoes, chopped
- ¼ cup water
- A pinch of salt and black pepper
- A pinch of cayenne pepper
- 1 pound shrimp, deveined

Directions:

Put sausage, onion, bell pepper and celery In your Crockpot. Add water, tomatoes, salt, pepper and cayenne, cover and cook on Low for 7 hours. Add shrimp, cover and cook on High for 30 minutes. Divide stew Into bowls and serve.
Enjoy!

Nutrition: calories 321, fat 4, fiber 7, carbs 8, protein 4

Tasty Seafood Stew

Preparation time: 10 minutes
Cooking time: 4 hours
Servings: 6

Ingredients:

- 28 ounces canned tomatoes, crushed
- 3 garlic cloves, minced
- 4 cups veggie stock
- 1 yellow onion, chopped
- 1 teaspoon basil, dried
- 1 teaspoon thyme, dried
- 1 teaspoon cilantro, dried
- A pinch of salt and black pepper
- ¼ teaspoon red pepper flakes
- A pinch of cayenne pepper
- 2 pounds mixed deveined shrimp, scallops and crab legs

Directions:

In your Crockpot, mix tomatoes with cloves, stock, onion, basil, thyme, cilantro, salt, pepper, pepper flakes and cayenne, cover and cook on High for 3 hours. Add mixed seafood, cover and cook on High for 1 more hour. Divide between bowls and serve right away.
Enjoy!

Nutrition: calories 251, fat 4, fiber 6, carbs 8, protein 12

Seafood Chowder

Preparation time: 10 minutes
Cooking time: 8 hours and 30 minutes
Servings: 4

Ingredients:

- 2 cups water
- ½ fennel bulb, chopped
- 1 yellow onion, chopped
- 2 bay leaves
- 1 tablespoon thyme, dried
- 1 celery rib, chopped
- A pinch of salt and black pepper
- A pinch of cayenne pepper
- 1 cup seafood stock
- 1 cup coconut milk
- 1 pounds salmon fillets, cubed
- 5 sea scallops, halved
- 24 shrimp, peeled and deveined
- ¼ cup parsley, chopped

Directions:

In your Crockpot, mix water with fennel, onion, bay leaves, thyme, celery, stock, cayenne, salt and black pepper, cover and cook on Low for 8 hours. Add salmon, coconut milk, scallops, shrimp and parsley, cover, cook on Low for 30 minutes more, ladle chowder Into bowls and serve.
Enjoy!

Nutrition: calories 354, fat 10, fiber 2, carbs 7, protein 12

Maple Salmon With Broccoli And Cauliflower

Preparation time: 10 minutes
Cooking time: 3 hours
Servings: 2

Ingredients:
- 2 medium salmon fillets, boneless
- A pinch of sea salt and black pepper
- 2 tablespoons coconut aminos
- 2 tablespoons maple syrup
- 16 ounces mixed broccoli and cauliflower florets
- 2 tablespoons lemon juice
- 1 teaspoon sesame seeds

Directions:
Put the cauliflower and broccoli florets In your Crockpot and top with salmon fillets. In a bowl, mix maple syrup with aminos and lemon juice and whisk really well. Pour this over salmon fillets, season with salt and black pepper, sprinkle sesame seeds on top and cook on Low for 3 hours. Divide everything between plates and serve right away.
Enjoy!

Nutrition: calories 230, fat 4, fiber 2, carbs 7, protein 6

Italian Shrimp

Preparation time: 10 minutes
Cooking time: 1 hour and 30 minutes
Servings: 4

Ingredients:
- 2 tablespoons olive oil
- ¼ cup chicken stock
- 1 tablespoon garlic, minced
- 2 tablespoons parsley, chopped
- Juice of ½ lemon
- A pinch of salt and black pepper to the taste
- 1 pound shrimp, peeled and deveined

Directions:
Put the oil In your Crockpot, add stock, garlic, parsley, lemon juice, salt and pepper and whisk. Add shrimp, stir, cover and cook on High for 1 hour and 30 minutes. Divide between bowls and serve.
Enjoy!

Nutrition: calories 140, fat 4, fiber 3, carbs 9, protein 3

Crock Pot Thai Pompano With Leeks

Preparation time: 10 minutes
Cooking time: 1 hour
Servings: 4

Ingredients:
- 1 pompano
- 2 tablespoons coconut aminos
- ¼ cup olive oil
- ¼ cup veggie stock
- 1 small ginger piece, grated
- 6 garlic cloves, minced
- 2 tablespoons Worcestershire sauce
- 1 bunch leeks, chopped
- 1 bunch cilantro, chopped

Directions:
Put the oil In your Crockpot, add leeks and top with the fish. In a bowl, mix stock with ginger, garlic, Worcestershire sauce, cilantro and aminos, whisk well, add to the pot, cover and cook on High for 1 hour. Divide fish between plates and serve with the sauce drizzled on top.
Enjoy!

Nutrition: calories 300, fat 8, fiber 2, carbs 8, protein 6

Spicy Tuna Loin

Preparation time: 10 minutes
Cooking time: 4 hours and 10 minutes
Servings: 2

Ingredients:
- ½ pound tuna loin, cubed
- 1 garlic clove, minced
- 4 jalapeno peppers, chopped
- 1 cup olive oil
- 3 red chili peppers, chopped
- 2 teaspoons black peppercorns, ground
- A pinch of salt and black pepper to the taste

Directions:
Put the oil In your Crockpot, add chili peppers, jalapenos, peppercorns, salt, pepper and garlic, whisk, cover and cook on Low for 4 hours. Add tuna cubes, cook on High for 10 minutes more, divide between plates and serve.
Enjoy!

Nutrition: calories 200, fat 4, fiber 3, carbs 7, protein 4

Crock Pot Braised Squid

Preparation time: 10 minutes
Cooking time: 7 hours
Servings: 4

Ingredients:
- 1 pound squid, cleaned and cut into rings
- 1/2 cup coconut sugar
- 1 small ginger piece, grated
- 1 garlic head, peeled and crushed
- 3 tablespoons coconut aminos
- 1/4 cup veggie stock
- 2 leeks stalks, chopped
- 2 bay leaves
- A pinch of salt and black pepper

Directions:
Put the squid In your Crockpot, add sugar, ginger, garlic, aminos, leeks, stock, black pepper and bay leaves, stir, cover and cook on Low for 8 hours. Divide between bowls and serve right away. Enjoy!

Nutrition: calories 190, fat 2, fiber 4, carbs 7, protein 5

Salmon With Cilantro Sauce

Preparation time: 10 minutes
Cooking time: 2 hours and 30 minutes
Servings: 4

Ingredients:
- 2 garlic cloves, minced
- 4 salmon fillets, boneless
- ¾ cup cilantro, chopped
- 3 tablespoons lime juice
- 1 tablespoon olive oil
- A pinch of salt and black pepper to the taste

Directions:
Grease your Crockpot with the oil, place salmon fillets inside skin side down, add garlic, cilantro, lime juice, salt and pepper, cover and cook on Low for2 hours and 30 minutes. Divide salmon fillets on plates, drizzle cilantro sauce from the Crockpot all over and serve.
Enjoy!

Nutrition: calories 180, fat 3, fiber 2, carbs 4, protein 8

Crock Pot Steamed Salmon

Preparation time: 10 minutes
Cooking time: 2 hours
Servings: 2

Ingredients:

- 1 medium salmon fillets
- A pinch of nutmeg, ground
- A pinch of cloves, ground
- A pinch of ginger powder
- A pinch of sea salt
- 2 teaspoons coconut sugar
- 1 teaspoon onion powder
- ¼ teaspoon chipotle chili powder
- ½ teaspoon cayenne pepper
- A pinch of salt and black pepper
- ½ teaspoon cinnamon powder
- ½ teaspoon thyme, dried

Directions:
In a bowl, mix salmon fillets with nutmeg, cloves, ginger, salt, coconut sugar, onion powder, chili powder, cayenne black pepper, cinnamon and thyme, rub, divide fish on 2 tin foil pieces, wrap, place In your Crockpot, cover and cook on Low for2 hours. Unwrap fish, divide between plates and serve with a side salad.
Enjoy!

Nutrition: calories 220, fat 4, fiber 2, carbs 7, protein 4

Creamy Clams

Preparation time: 10 minutes
Cooking time: 6 hours
Servings: 4

Ingredients:

- 21 ounces canned clams, chopped
- 1/3 cup coconut milk
- 4 eggs, whisked
- 2 tablespoons olive oil
- 1/3 cup green bell pepper, chopped
- ½ cup yellow onion, chopped
- Black pepper to the taste
- A pinch of sea salt

Directions:
Put clams In your Crockpot. In a bowl, mix milk, eggs, oil, onion, bell pepper, a pinch of salt and black pepper, whisk and add over clams. Stir, cover, cook on Low for 6 hours, divide between bowls and serve.
Enjoy!

Nutrition: calories 190, fat 4, fiber 2, carbs 6, protein 7

Ketogenic Crock Pot Side Dishes

Mexican Veggie Mix

Preparation time: 10 minutes
Cooking time: 2 hours
Servings: 4

Ingredients:
- 3 cups carrots, shredded
- 1 celery stalk, chopped
- ½ green cabbage head, shredded
- 2 zucchinis, chopped
- 1 sweet onion, chopped
- 4 tomatoes, chopped
- 2 tablespoons tomato paste
- 5 garlic cloves, minced
- 2 jalapenos, chopped
- 1 cup cilantro, chopped
- 3 cups chicken stock
- 1 tablespoon cumin, ground
- 1 tablespoon chili powder
- A drizzle of olive oil
- A pinch of salt and black pepper

Directions:
Grease your Crockpot with the oil and arrange carrots, celery, cabbage, zucchinis, onion and tomatoes In the pot. Add tomato paste, garlic, jalapenos, cilantro, stock, cumin, chili powder, salt and pepper, cover and cook on Low for 2 hours. Divide between plates and serve as a side dish. Enjoy!

Nutrition: calories 211, fat 3, fiber 3, carbs 6, protein 8

Fresh Veggie Side Dish

Preparation time: 10 minutes
Cooking time: 3 hours
Servings: 4

Ingredients:
- 2 cups okra, sliced
- 1 and ½ cups red onion, roughly chopped
- 1 cup cherry tomatoes, halved
- 2 and ½ cups zucchini, sliced
- 2 cups red and yellow bell peppers, sliced
- 1 cup white mushrooms, sliced
- ½ cup olive oil
- ½ cup balsamic vinegar
- 2 tablespoons basil, chopped
- 1 tablespoon thyme, chopped

Directions:
In your Crockpot, mix okra with onion, tomatoes, zucchini, bell peppers, mushrooms, basil and thyme. In a bowl mix oil with vinegar, whisk well, add to the pot, cover and cook on High for 3 hours. Divide between plates and serve as a side dish.
Enjoy!

Nutrition: calories 233, fat 12, fiber 4, carbs 8, protein 4

Spinach And Carrots Mix

Preparation time: 10 minutes
Cooking time: 4 hours
Servings: 6

Ingredients:
- 5 carrots, sliced
- 2 garlic cloves, minced
- 1 yellow onion, chopped
- A pinch of salt and black pepper
- ½ teaspoon oregano, dried
- 5 ounces baby spinach
- 2 and ½ cups veggie stock
- 2 teaspoons lemon peel, grated
- 3 tablespoons lemon juice
- 1 avocado, pitted, peeled and chopped
- ¾ cup goat cheese, crumbled

Directions:
In your Crockpot, mix onion, carrots, garlic, salt, pepper, oregano and stock, stir, cover and cook on High for 4 hours. Add spinach, lemon juice and lemon peel, stir, leave aside for 5 minutes, divide between plates, sprinkle goat cheese and avocado on top and serve as a side dish.
Enjoy!

Nutrition: calories 219, fat 8, fiber 4, carbs 8, protein 17

Cauliflower And Broccoli Fresh Mix

Preparation time: 10 minutes
Cooking time: 3 hours
Servings: 10

Ingredients:
- 4 cups broccoli florets
- 4 cups cauliflower florets
- 14 ounces tomato paste
- 1 yellow onion, chopped
- 1 teaspoon thyme, dried
- Salt and black pepper to the taste
- ½ cup almonds, sliced

Directions:
In your Crockpot, mix broccoli with cauliflower, tomato paste, onion, thyme, salt and pepper, toss, cover and cook on High for 3 hours. Divide between plates and serve as a side dish with almonds sprinkled on top.
Enjoy!

Nutrition: calories 177, fat 12, fiber 2, carbs 7, protein 7

Special Cauliflower Rice Mix

Preparation time: 10 minutes
Cooking time: 6 hours
Servings: 12

Ingredients:

- 2 cups veggie stock
- 2 and ½ cups cauliflower rice
- 1 cup carrot, shredded
- 4 ounces mushrooms, sliced
- 2 tablespoons olive oil
- 2 teaspoons marjoram, dried and crushed
- Salt and black pepper to the taste
- 2/3 cup dried cherries
- 2/3 cup green onions, chopped

Directions:
In your Crockpot, mix stock with cauliflower rice, carrot, mushrooms, oil, marjoram, salt, pepper, cherries and green onions, toss, cover and cook on Low for 6 hours. Divide between plates and serve as a side dish.
Enjoy!

Nutrition: calories 169, fat 5, fiber 3, carbs 8, protein 5

Rustic Mashed Cauliflower

Preparation time: 10 minutes
Cooking time: 4 hours
Servings: 6

Ingredients:

- 6 garlic cloves, peeled
- 1 big cauliflower head, florets separated
- 1 bay leaf
- 1 cup coconut milk
- 3 cups veggie stock
- 1 tablespoons olive oil
- Salt and black pepper to the taste

Directions:
In your Crockpot, mix cauliflower with stock, bay leaf, garlic, salt and pepper, cover and cook on High for 4 hours. Drain cauliflower mix, return to your Crockpot and mash using a potato masher. Add oil and coconut milk, whisk well, divide between plates and serve as a side dish. Enjoy!

Nutrition: calories 135, fat 5, fiber 1, carbs 7, protein 3

Carrots And Parsnips Mix

Preparation time: 10 minutes
Cooking time: 4 hours
Servings: 10

Ingredients:

- 1 pound parsnips, cut into medium chunks
- 2 pounds carrots, cut into medium chunks
- 2 tablespoons lemon peel, grated
- 1 cup veggie stock
- A pinch of salt and black pepper
- 3 tablespoons olive oil
- ¼ cup parsley, chopped

Directions:

In your Crockpot, mix parsnips with carrots, lemon peel, stock, salt, pepper, oil and parsley, cover and cook on High for 4 hours. Divide between plates and serve as a side dish.
Enjoy!

Nutrition: calories 159, fat 4, fiber 4, carbs 6, protein 2

Squash And Spinach Mix

Preparation time: 10 minutes
Cooking time: 3 hours and 30 minutes
Servings: 10

Ingredients:

- 10 ounces spinach, torn
- 2 pounds butternut squash, peeled and cubed
- 1 yellow onion, chopped
- 2 cups veggie stock
- ½ cup water
- A pinch of salt and black pepper
- 3 garlic cloves, minced

Directions:

In your Crockpot, mix squash with spinach, onion, stock, water, salt, pepper and garlic, toss, cover and cook on High for 3 hours and 30 minutes. Divide squash mix on plates and serve as a side dish.
Enjoy!

Nutrition: calories 196, fat 3, fiber 7, carbs 8, protein 7

Fall Veggie Mix

Preparation time: 10 minutes
Cooking time: 8 hours
Servings: 6

Ingredients:

- 2 tablespoons olive oil
- 2 tablespoons rosemary, chopped
- A pinch of salt and black pepper
- 2 cups cherry tomatoes, halved
- 2 garlic cloves, minced
- 1 pound cauliflower, florets separated
- 12 small baby carrots, peeled
- 28 ounces veggie stock
- 1 yellow onion, cut into medium wedges
- 4 cups baby spinach
- 8 ounces zucchini, sliced

Directions:

In your Crockpot, mix oil, rosemary, salt, pepper, cherry tomatoes, garlic, cauliflower, baby carrots, onion, zucchini, spinach and stock, stir, cover and cook on Low for 8 hours. Divide everything between plates and serve as a side dish.
Enjoy!

Nutrition: calories 273, fat 7, fiber 5, carbs 8, protein 12

Eggplant And Kale Mix

Preparation time: 10 minutes
Cooking time:2 hours
Servings: 6

Ingredients:

- 14 ounces canned roasted tomatoes and garlic
- 4 cups eggplant, cubed
- 1 yellow bell pepper, chopped
- 1 red onion, cut into medium wedges
- 4 cups kale leaves
- 2 tablespoons olive oil
- 1 teaspoon mustard
- 3 tablespoons red vinegar
- 1 garlic clove, minced
- A pinch of salt and black pepper
- ½ cup basil, chopped

Directions:

In your Crockpot, mix the eggplant cubes with tomatoes, bell pepper and onion, toss, cover and cook on High for2 hours. Add kale, toss, cover Crockpot and leave aside for now. Meanwhile, In a bowl, mix oil with vinegar, mustard, garlic, salt and pepper and whisk well. Add this and basil over eggplant mix, toss, divide between plates and serve as a side dish.
Enjoy!

Nutrition: calories 251, fat 9, fiber 6, carbs 7, protein 8

Brussels Sprouts And Onions

Preparation time: 10 minutes
Cooking time: 3 hours
Servings: 10

Ingredients:
- 1 cup red onion, chopped
- 2 pounds Brussels sprouts, trimmed and halved
- A pinch of salt and black pepper
- ¼ cup apple juice
- 3 tablespoons olive oil
- ¼ cup maple syrup
- 1 tablespoon thyme, chopped

Directions:
In your Crockpot, mix sprouts with onion, salt, pepper and apple juice, toss, cover and cook on Low for 3 hours. In a bowl, mix maple syrup with oil and thyme, whisk really well, add over sprouts mix, toss, divide between plates and serve as a side dish.
Enjoy!

Nutrition: calories 100, fat 4, fiber 4, carbs 8, protein 3

Cabbage And Apples Side Dish

Preparation time: 10 minutes
Cooking time: 6 hours
Servings: 4

Ingredients:
- 1 onion, sliced
- 1 cabbage, shredded
- 2 apples, peeled, cored and roughly chopped
- A pinch of salt and black pepper
- 1 cup apple juice
- ½ cup chicken stock
- 3 tablespoons mustard
- 1 tablespoon coconut oil, melted

Directions:
Grease your Crockpot with the coconut oil and place apples, cabbage and onions Inside. In a bowl, mix stock with mustard, salt, black pepper and the apple juice, whisk well, add to Crockpot, cover and cook on Low for 6 hours. Divide between plates and serve right away as a side dish.
Enjoy!

Nutrition: calories 200, fat 4, fiber 2, carbs 8, protein 6

Simple Mushrooms Caps Side Dish

Preparation time: 10 minutes
Cooking time: 4 hours
Servings: 4

Ingredients:
- 2 bay leaves
- 4 garlic cloves, minced
- 24 ounces white mushroom caps
- ¼ teaspoon thyme dried
- ½ teaspoon basil, dried
- ½ teaspoon oregano, dried
- 1 cup veggie stock
- A pinch of salt and black pepper
- 2 tablespoons olive oil
- 2 tablespoons parsley, chopped

Directions:
Grease your Crockpot with the oil, add mushrooms, garlic, bay leaves, thyme, basil, oregano, black pepper and stock, cover and cook on Low for 4 hours. Divide between plates and serve with parsley sprinkled on top as a side dish.
Enjoy!

Nutrition: calories 122, fat 6, fiber 1, carbs 8, protein 5

Zucchini And Squash Side Dish

Preparation time: 10 minutes
Cooking time: 6 hours
Servings: 6

Ingredients:
- 2 cups zucchinis, sliced
- 1 teaspoon Italian seasoning
- Black pepper to the taste
- 2 cups yellow squash, peeled and cut into wedges
- 1 teaspoon garlic powder
- 2 tablespoons olive oil
- A pinch of salt and black pepper

Directions:
Grease your Crockpot with the oil, add zucchini, squash, Italian seasoning, black pepper, salt and garlic powder, toss well, cover and cook on Low for 6 hours. Divide between plates and serve as a side dish.
Enjoy!

Nutrition: calories 100, fat 2, fiber 4, carbs 8, protein 5

Cheesy Green Beans

Preparation time: 10 minutes
Cooking time: 3 hours and 30 minutes
Servings: 4

Ingredients:

- 2/3 cup parmesan, grated
- 1 egg
- 12 ounces green beans
- Salt and black pepper to the taste
- ½ teaspoon garlic powder
- ¼ teaspoon sweet paprika

Directions:

In a bowl, mix the egg with parmesan with salt, pepper, garlic powder and paprika and whisk. Put green beans In your Crockpot, add egg and parmesan mix over them, toss well, cover and cook on Low for 3 hours and 30 minutes. Divide between plates and serve as a side dish. Enjoy!

Nutrition: calories 114, fat 5, fiber 6, carbs 8, protein 9

Herbed Mushrooms Mix

Preparation time: 10 minutes
Cooking time: 3 hours
Servings: 4

Ingredients:

- 12 ounces Portobello mushrooms, sliced
- Salt and black pepper to the taste
- ½ teaspoon basil, dried
- 2 tablespoons olive oil
- ½ teaspoon tarragon, dried
- ½ teaspoon rosemary, dried
- ½ teaspoon thyme, dried
- 2 tablespoons balsamic vinegar

Directions:

In a bowl, mix oil with vinegar, salt, pepper, rosemary, tarragon, basil and thyme and whisk well. Add mushroom slices, toss to coat well, transfer to your Crockpot, cover and cook on Low for 3 hours. Divide between plates and serve as a side dish. Enjoy!

Nutrition: calories 80, fat 4, fiber 4, carbs 8, protein 4

Brussels Sprouts And Bacon

Preparation time: 10 minutes
Cooking time: 6 hours
Servings: 4

Ingredients:

- 8 bacon strips, chopped
- 1 pound Brussels sprouts, trimmed and halved
- Salt and black pepper to the taste
- A pinch of cumin, ground
- A pinch of red pepper, crushed
- 2 tablespoons olive oil

Directions:
In a bowl, mix Brussels sprouts with salt, pepper, cumin, red pepper and oil, toss to coat, transfer to your Crockpot, add bacon on top, cover and cook on Low for 6 hours. Divide between plates and serve as a side dish.
Enjoy!

Nutrition: calories 256, fat 12, fiber 6, carbs 8, protein 15

Creamy Spinach

Preparation time: 10 minutes
Cooking time: 3 hours
Servings: 2

Ingredients:

- 2 garlic cloves, minced
- 8 ounces spinach leaves
- A drizzle of olive oil
- Salt and black pepper to the taste
- 4 tablespoons coconut cream
- 2 tablespoons parmesan cheese, grated

Directions:
Grease your Crockpot with the oil, add garlic, spinach, salt, pepper and coconut cream, toss, cover and cook on Low for 3 hours. Add parmesan, toss until it melts, divide between plates and serve as a side dish.
Enjoy!

Nutrition: calories 133, fat 10, fiber 4, carbs 4, protein 2

Okra And Mint

Preparation time: 10 minutes
Cooking time: 3 hours
Servings: 4

Ingredients:

- 1 pound okra, sliced
- Salt and black pepper to the taste
- 1 tablespoon mint, chopped
- 2 teaspoons olive oil
- 2 tablespoons chicken stock
- 3 green onions, chopped
- 1 garlic clove, minced

Directions:
Grease your Crockpot with the oil, add okra, salt, pepper, mint, stock, garlic and green onions, toss, cover and cook on Low for 3 hours. Divide between plates and serve as a side dish.
Enjoy!

Nutrition: calories 70, fat 1, fiber 1, carbs 4, protein 6

Napa Cabbage Mix

Preparation time: 10 minutes
Cooking time:2 hours
Servings: 6

Ingredients:

- 1 pound napa cabbage, chopped
- A pinch of salt and black pepper
- 1 carrot, julienned
- 2 tablespoons veggie stock
- ½ cup radish, sliced
- 3 garlic cloves, minced
- 3 green onion stalks, chopped
- 1 tablespoon coconut aminos
- 3 tablespoons chili flakes
- 1 tablespoon olive oil
- ½ Inch ginger, grated

Directions:
In your Crockpot, mix cabbage with salt, pepper, carrot, stock, radish, garlic, green onions, aminos, chili flakes, oil and ginger, toss, cover and cook on High for2 hours. Divide between plates and serve as a side dish.
Enjoy!

Nutrition: calories 100, fat 3, fiber 4, carbs 5, protein 2

Garlicky Swiss Chard

Preparation time: 10 minutes
Cooking time: 2 hours
Servings: 4

Ingredients:

- 2 tablespoons olive oil
- 3 tablespoons lemon juice
- ½ cup chicken stock
- 4 bacon slices, chopped
- 2 bunches Swiss chard, roughly torn
- ½ teaspoon garlic paste
- Salt and black pepper to the taste

Directions:
In your Crockpot, mix oil with chard, bacon, stock, lemon juice, garlic paste, salt and pepper, toss, cover and cook on High for 2 hours. Divide between plates and serve as a side dish.
Enjoy

Nutrition: calories 160, fat 7, fiber 3, carbs 6, protein 4

Mushroom And Arugula Mix

Preparation time: 10 minutes
Cooking time: 2 hours
Servings: 4

Ingredients:

- 2 tablespoons olive oil
- Salt and black pepper to the taste
- 1 pound cremini mushrooms, roughly chopped
- 4 tablespoons veggie stock
- 4 bunches arugula
- 8 slices prosciutto, chopped
- 2 tablespoons balsamic vinegar
- 8 sun dried tomatoes, chopped
- 1 tablespoon parsley, chopped

Directions:
In your Crockpot, mix mushrooms with oil, salt, pepper, stock, prosciutto, vinegar and tomatoes, toss, cover and cook on High for 2 hours. Add arugula and parsley, toss, leave aside for a few minutes, divide between plates and serve as a side dish.
Enjoy!

Nutrition: calories 200, fat 3, fiber 2, carbs 5, protein 6

Red Chard Mix

Preparation time: 10 minutes
Cooking time: 2 hours
Servings: 4

Ingredients:

- 2 tablespoons olive oil
- 2 bunches red chard, roughly chopped
- 3 tablespoons veggie stock
- 2 tablespoons capers
- 1 yellow onion, chopped
- Juice of 1 lemon
- Salt and black pepper to the taste
- 1 teaspoon stevia
- ¼ cup kalamata olives, pitted and chopped

Directions:
Grease your Crockpot with the oil, add red chard, stock, onion, lemon juice, salt, pepper, stevia and olives, toss a bit, cover and cook on High for2 hours. Add capers, divide between plates and serve as a side dish.
Enjoy!

Nutrition: calories 123, fat 4, fiber 3, carbs 4, protein 5

Kale Side Dish

Preparation time: 10 minutes
Cooking time: 2 hours
Servings: 4

Ingredients:

- 1 cup chicken stock
- A pinch of salt and black pepper
- 1 big kale bunch, roughly torn
- 1 tablespoon balsamic vinegar
- 1/3 cup almonds, toasted
- 3 garlic cloves, minced
- 1 small yellow onion, chopped
- 2 tablespoons olive oil

Directions:
Grease your Crockpot with the oil, add kale, stock, vinegar, onion, garlic, salt and pepper, toss, cover and cook on High for2 hours. Add almonds, toss and serve as a side dish.
Enjoy!

Nutrition: calories 140, fat 6, fiber 3, carbs 5, protein 3

Hungarian Cabbage Side Dish

Preparation time: 10 minutes
Cooking time: 2 hours and 30 minutes
Servings: 4

Ingredients:
- 1 and ½ pound green cabbage, shredded
- Salt and black pepper to the taste
- 3 tablespoons olive oil
- 1 cup veggie stock
- ¼ teaspoon sweet paprika

Directions:
Grease your Crockpot with the oil, add cabbage, salt, pepper, paprika and stock, cover and cook on High for 2 hours and 30 minutes. Divide between plates and serve as a side dish.
Enjoy!

Nutrition: calories 170, fat 4, fiber 2, carbs 5, protein 5

Mushrooms Winter Mix

Preparation time: 10 minutes
Cooking time: 3 hours
Servings: 4

Ingredients:
- 4 tablespoons avocado oil
- 3 tablespoons veggie stock
- 1 teaspoon garlic powder
- 16 ounces baby mushrooms
- Salt and black pepper to the taste
- 3 tablespoons onion, dried
- 3 tablespoons parsley flakes

Directions:
Grease your Crockpot with the oil, add mushrooms, stock, garlic powder, salt, pepper, dried onion and parsley flakes, cover and cook on High for 3 hours. Divide between plates and serve as a side dish.
Enjoy!

Nutrition: calories 192, fat 6, fiber 5, carbs 6, protein 2

Balsamic Swiss Chard With Pine Nuts And Raisins

Preparation time: 10 minutes
Cooking time: 2 hours
Servings: 4

Ingredients:

- 1 bunch Swiss chard, cut into strips
- 2 tablespoons olive oil
- 1 tablespoon balsamic vinegar
- A pinch of salt and black pepper
- 1 small yellow onion, chopped
- ¼ teaspoon red pepper flakes
- ¼ cup pine nuts, toasted
- ¼ cup raisins

Directions:
Grease your Crockpot with the oil, add Swiss chard, vinegar, salt, pepper, onion and pepper flakes, cover and cook on High for 2 hours. Add raisins and pine nuts, toss, divide between plates and serve as a side dish.
Enjoy!

Nutrition: calories 120, fat 2, fiber 1, carbs 7, protein 4

Balsamic Spinach And Chard

Preparation time: 10 minutes
Cooking time: 2 hours and 20 minutes
Servings: 4

Ingredients:

- 1 yellow onion, sliced
- 4 tablespoons pine nuts, toasted
- 2 tablespoons olive oil
- 6 garlic cloves, chopped
- ¼ cup balsamic vinegar
- 2 and ½ cups baby spinach
- 2 and ½ cups Swiss chard, roughly torn
- Salt and black pepper to the taste
- A pinch of nutmeg

Directions:
Grease your Crockpot with the oil, add onion, garlic, spinach, chard, salt, pepper, nutmeg and vinegar, toss a bit, cover and cook on High for 2 hours and 30 minutes. Add pine nuts, toss, divide between plates and serve as a side dish.
Enjoy!

Nutrition: calories 140, fat 1, fiber 2, carbs 3, protein 3

Cherry Tomatoes Side Dish

Preparation time: 10 minutes
Cooking time:2 hours
Servings: 6

Ingredients:
- 1 jalapeno pepper, chopped
- 4 garlic cloves, minced
- Salt and black pepper to the taste
- 2 pounds cherry tomatoes, halved
- 1 yellow onion, cut into wedges
- ¼ cup olive oil
- ½ teaspoon oregano, dried
- 1 and ½ cups chicken stock
- ¼ cup basil, chopped
- ½ cup parmesan, grated

Directions:
Grease your Crockpot with the oil, add tomatoes, jalapeno, garlic, salt, pepper, onion, oregano and stock, toss a bit, cover and cook on High for2 hours. Add parmesan and basil, toss, divide between plates and serve as a side dish.
Enjoy!

Nutrition: calories 120, fat 2, fiber 3, carbs 5, protein 4

Squash Mash

Preparation time: 10 minutes
Cooking time: 4 hours
Servings: 4

Ingredients:
- ½ cup stock
- 2 acorn squash, peeled, roughly cubed and seeds removed
- Salt and black pepper to the taste
- ¼ teaspoon baking soda
- 2 tablespoons avocado oil
- ½ teaspoon nutmeg, ground
- 2 tablespoons stevia

Directions:
In your Crockpot, mix squash with stock, salt, pepper and stevia, cover and cook on Low for 4 hours. Mash squash using a potato masher, add oil, baking soda and nutmeg, whisk well, divide between plates and serve as a side dish.
Enjoy!

Nutrition: calories 152, fat 3, fiber 2, carbs 4, protein 9

Red Chard And Capers

Preparation time: 10 minutes
Cooking time: 3 hours
Servings: 4

Ingredients:
- 2 tablespoons olive oil
- 2 tablespoons chicken stock
- 1 yellow onion, chopped
- 2 tablespoons capers
- Juice of 1 lemon
- Salt and black pepper to the taste
- 1 teaspoon palm sugar
- 1 bunch red chard, chopped
- ¼ cup kalamata olives, pitted and chopped

Directions:
Grease your Crockpot with the oil, add chard, stock, onion, salt, pepper, lemon juice and palm sugar, toss, cover and cook on Low for 3 hours. Add olives and capers, toss, divide between plates and serve as a side dish.
Enjoy!

Nutrition: calories 119, fat 7, fiber 3, carbs 7, protein 2

Balsamic Kale

Preparation time: 10 minutes
Cooking time: 4 hours
Servings: 4

Ingredients:
- 2 cups veggie stock
- 1 tablespoon balsamic vinegar
- 1/3 cup almonds, toasted
- 3 garlic cloves, minced
- 1 bunch kale, steamed and chopped
- 1 small yellow onion, chopped
- 2 tablespoons olive oil

Directions:
Grease your Crockpot with the oil, add kale, stock, vinegar, garlic and onion, cover and cook on Low for 4 hours. Add almonds, toss, divide between plates and serve as a side dish.
Enjoy!

Nutrition: calories 170, fat 11, fiber 3, carbs 7, protein 7

Simple Broccoli Side Dish

Preparation time: 5 minutes
Cooking time: 4 hours
Servings: 6

Ingredients:
- 31 oz broccoli, florets separated
- 1 cup chicken stock
- 5 lemon slices
- Salt and black pepper to the taste

Directions:
In your Crockpot, mix broccoli with stock, lemon slices, salt and pepper, cover and cook on Low for 4 hours. Divide broccoli between plates and serve as a side dish.
Enjoy!

Nutrition: calories 82, fat 1, fiber 2, carbs 6, protein 3

Fast And Creamy Fennel Mix

Preparation time: 5 minutes
Cooking time: 3 hours
Servings: 3

Ingredients:
- 2 big fennel bulbs, sliced
- 2 tablespoons olive oil
- 1 tablespoon coconut flour
- 2 cups coconut milk
- ¼ teaspoon nutmeg, ground
- Salt and black pepper to the taste.

Directions:
Grease your Crockpot with the oil, add fennel, coconut milk, flour, nutmeg, salt and pepper, toss, cover and cook on High for 3 hours. Divide between plates and serve as a side dish.
Enjoy!

Nutrition: calories 121, fat 2, fiber 3, carbs 6, protein 12

Colored Bell Peppers Mix

Preparation time: 10 minutes
Cooking time: 3 hours
Servings: 4

Ingredients:

- 2 yellow bell peppers, thinly sliced
- 1 green bell pepper, thinly sliced
- 2 red bell peppers, thinly sliced
- 2 tomatoes, chopped
- 2 garlic cloves, minced
- 4 tablespoons chicken stock
- 1 red onion, thinly sliced
- Salt and black pepper to the taste
- 1 bunch parsley, finely chopped
- A drizzle of olive oil

Directions:
Grease your Crockpot with the oil and add yellow, green and red bell peppers. Also add stock, tomatoes, garlic, onion, salt and pepper, cover and cook on High for 3 hours. Add parsley, toss, divide between plates and serve as a side dish.
Enjoy!

Nutrition: calories 152, fat 3, fiber 3, carbs 5, protein 4

Broccoli And Tomatoes Mix

Preparation time: 10 minutes
Cooking time: 4 hours
Servings: 4

Ingredients:

- 1 broccoli head, florets separated
- 2 teaspoons coriander, ground
- A drizzle of olive oil
- 1 yellow onion, chopped
- Salt and black pepper to the taste
- A pinch of red pepper, crushed
- 1 small ginger piece, chopped
- 1 garlic clove, minced
- 28 ounces canned tomatoes, pureed

Directions:
Grease your Crockpot with the oil, add broccoli, coriander, onion, salt, pepper, red pepper, ginger, garlic and tomatoes, toss a bit, cover and cook on Low for 4 hours. Divide between plates and serve as a side dish.
Enjoy!

Nutrition: calories 150, fat 4, fiber 2, carbs 5, protein 12

Bok Choy And Bacon Mix

Preparation time: 10 minutes
Cooking time:2 hours
Servings: 2

Ingredients:
- 2 garlic cloves, minced
- 2 cup bok choy, chopped
- 4 tablespoons chicken stock
- 2 bacon slices, chopped
- Salt and black pepper to the taste
- A drizzle of avocado oil

Directions:
Grease your Crockpot with the oil, add bok choy, stock, garlic, bacon, salt and pepper, cover and cook on High for2 hours. Divide between plates and serve as a side dish.
Enjoy!

Nutrition: calories 50, fat 1, fiber 4, carbs 8, protein 8

Creamy Celery Side Dish

Preparation time: 10 minutes
Cooking time: 4 hours
Servings: 8

Ingredients:
- 26 ounces celery leaves and stalks, chopped
- 1 tablespoon onion flakes
- Salt and black pepper to the taste
- 3 teaspoons fenugreek powder
- 3 tablespoons veggie stock
- 6 ounces coconut cream

Directions:
 In your Crockpot, mix celery with onion flakes, salt, pepper, fenugreek, stock and cream, cover and cook on Low for 4 hours. Divide between plates and serve as a side dish.
Enjoy!

Nutrition: calories 140, fat 2, fiber 1, carbs 5, protein 10

Stewed Celery Mix

Preparation time: 10 minutes
Cooking time: 4 hours
Servings: 6

Ingredients:
- 1 celery bunch, roughly chopped
- 1 yellow onion, chopped
- 1 bunch green onion, chopped
- 4 garlic cloves, minced
- Salt and black pepper to the taste
- 1 parsley bunch, chopped
- 2 mint bunches, chopped
- 2 cups veggie stock
- 4 tablespoons olive oil

Directions:
Grease your Crockpot with the oil, add celery, onion, green onion, garlic, salt, pepper and stock, cover and cook on Low for 3 hours and 30 minutes. Add parsley and mint, cover and cook on Low for 30 minutes more. Divide between plates and serve as a side dish.
Enjoy!

Nutrition: calories 170, fat 7, fiber 4, carbs 6, protein 10

Lemony Collard Greens

Preparation time: 10 minutes
Cooking time: 3 hours
Servings: 4

Ingredients:
- 2 garlic cloves, minced
- ½ cup veggie stock
- 2 and ½ pounds collard greens, chopped
- 1 teaspoon lemon juice
- 1 tablespoon olive oil
- Salt and black pepper to the taste

Directions:
Grease your Crockpot with the oil, add greens, garlic, stock, lemon juice, salt and pepper, cover and cook on Low for 3 hours. Divide between plates and serve as a side dish.
Enjoy!

Nutrition: calories 151, fat 6, fiber 3, carbs 7, protein 8

Collard Greens, Bacon And Tomatoes

Preparation time: 10 minutes
Cooking time: 3 hours
Servings: 4

Ingredients:
- 1 pound collard greens
- 3 bacon strips, chopped
- ¼ cup cherry tomatoes, halved
- A drizzle of olive oil
- 1 tablespoon balsamic vinegar
- 2 tablespoons chicken stock
- Salt and black pepper to the taste

Directions:
Grease your Crockpot with the oil and add bacon on the bottom. Add collard greens, tomatoes, vinegar, stock, salt and pepper, cover and cook on Low for 3 hours. Divide between plates and serve as a side dish.
Enjoy!

Nutrition: calories 120, fat 8, fiber 1, carbs 3, protein 7

Mustard Greens And Garlic

Preparation time: 5 minutes
Cooking time: 2 hours
Servings: 4

Ingredients:
- 2 garlic cloves, minced
- 1 pound mustard greens, roughly torn
- 1 tablespoon olive oil
- ½ cup yellow onion, sliced
- Salt and black pepper to the taste
- ¼ cup veggie stock
- ¼ teaspoon avocado oil

Directions:
Grease Crockpot with the olive oil, add garlic, greens, onion, salt, pepper and stock, cover and cook on High for 2 hours. Add avocado oil, toss, divide between plates and serve as a side dish.
Enjoy!

Nutrition: calories 120, fat 3, fiber 1, carbs 3, protein 6

Cheesy Collard Greens

Preparation time: 10 minutes
Cooking time: 2 hours and 40 minutes
Servings: 6

Ingredients:

- 1 tablespoon chipotle In adobo, mashed
- 6 eggs, whisked
- 3 tablespoons olive oil
- 1 yellow onion, chopped
- 2 garlic cloves, minced
- 6 bacon slices, chopped
- 3 bunches collard greens, chopped
- ½ cup chicken stock
- Salt and black pepper to the taste
- 1 tablespoon lime juice
- 1 tablespoon cheddar cheese

Directions:
Add the oil to your Crockpot and arrange chipotle on the bottom. Add onion, garlic, bacon, collard greens, stock, salt, pepper, lime juice and whisked eggs, toss, cover and cook on High for 2 hours and 40 minutes. Add cheese, toss until it melts, divide between plates and serve as a side dish.
Enjoy!

Nutrition: calories 245, fat 13, fiber 1, carbs 5, protein 12

Spring Green Mix

Preparation time: 10 minutes
Cooking time: 4 hours
Servings: 4

Ingredients:

- 2 cups mustard greens, chopped
- 2 cups collard greens, chopped
- 2 cups veggie stock
- 1 yellow onion, chopped
- Salt and black pepper to the taste
- 2 tablespoons coconut aminos
- 2 teaspoons ginger, grated

Directions:
In your Crockpot, mix mustard greens with collard greens, stock, onion, salt, pepper, aminos and ginger, toss, cover and cook on Low for 4 hours. Divide between plates and serve as a side dish.
Enjoy!

Nutrition: calories 140, fat 2, fiber 1, carbs 3, protein 12

Easy Asparagus

Preparation time: 10 minutes
Cooking time: 2 hours and 30 minutes
Servings: 3

Ingredients:
- 10 ounces asparagus spears, cut into medium pieces and steamed
- Salt and black pepper to the taste
- 2 tablespoons parmesan, grated
- 1/3 cup Monterey jack cheese, shredded
- 2 tablespoons mustard
- 4 ounces coconut cream
- 3 tablespoons bacon, cooked and crumbled

Directions:
In your Crockpot, mix asparagus with salt, pepper, mustard, cream and bacon, cover and cook on High for 2 hours and 30 minutes. Add Monterey jack and parmesan cheese, toss until cheese melts, divide between plates and serve as a side dish.
Enjoy!

Nutrition: calories 206, fat 13, fiber 2, carbs 5, protein 13

Spanish Spinach Mix

Preparation time: 10 minutes
Cooking time: 3 hours
Servings: 4

Ingredients:
- 1 yellow onion, sliced
- 3 tablespoons avocado oil
- ¼ cup raisins
- ¼ cup chicken stock
- 6 garlic cloves, chopped
- ¼ cup pine nuts, toasted
- ¼ cup balsamic vinegar
- ½ teaspoon nutmeg, ground
- 5 cups mixed spinach and chard
- Salt and black pepper to the taste

Directions:
Grease your Crockpot with the oil, add onion, stock, garlic, vinegar, nutmeg, spinach, salt and pepper, toss a bit, cover and cook on High for 3 hours. Add raisins and pine nuts, toss, divide between plates and serve as a side dish.
Enjoy!

Nutrition: calories 120, fat 1, fiber 2, carbs 3, protein 6

Squash And Swiss Chard Mix

Preparation time: 10 minutes
Cooking time: 2 hours
Servings: 4

Ingredients:

- 1 red onion, chopped
- 1 bunch Swiss chard, roughly chopped
- 1 yellow squash, cubed
- 1 zucchini, cubed
- 1 green bell pepper, chopped
- Salt and black pepper to the taste
- 6 carrots, chopped
- 4 cups tomatoes, chopped
- 1 cup cauliflower florets, chopped
- 2 cups chicken stock
- 3 ounces canned tomato paste
- 1 pound sausage, chopped
- 2 garlic cloves, minced
- 2 teaspoons thyme, chopped
- 1 teaspoon rosemary, dried
- 1 tablespoon fennel, minced
- ½ teaspoon red pepper flake

Directions:
Heat up a pan over medium- high heat, add sausage and garlic, stir and cook until it browns and transfer along with its juices to your Crockpot. Add onion, Swiss chard, squash, bell pepper, zucchini, carrots, tomatoes, cauliflower, tomato paste, stock, thyme, fennel, rosemary, pepper flakes, salt and pepper, stir, cover and cook on High for 2 hours. Divide between plates and serve as a side dish.
Enjoy!

Nutrition: calories 190, fat 8, fiber 2, carbs 4, protein 9

Simple Cherry Tomatoes And Onion Mix

Preparation time: 10 minutes
Cooking time: 4 hours
Servings: 5

Ingredients:

- 4 garlic cloves, minced
- 2 pounds cherry tomatoes, halved
- 1 red onion, cut into wedges
- Salt and black pepper to the taste
- 3 tablespoons avocado oil
- ½ teaspoon basil, dried
- 1 and ½ cups veggie stock
- ¼ cup parsley, chopped
- ½ cup goat cheese, crumbled

Directions:
Grease your Crockpot with the oil, add garlic, tomatoes, onion wedges, salt, pepper, basil and stock, cover and cook on Low for 4 hours. Divide between plates and serve as a side dish with parsley and goat cheese crumbled on top.
Enjoy!

Nutrition: calories 140, fat 2, fiber 2, carbs 5, protein 8

Creamy Eggplant And Tomatoes

Preparation time: 10 minutes
Cooking time: 5 hours
Servings: 4

Ingredients:

- 4 tomatoes, cut into wedges
- 1 teaspoon garlic, minced
- ¼ yellow onion, chopped
- Salt and black pepper to the taste
- 1 cup chicken stock
- 1 bay leaf
- ½ cup coconut cream
- 2 tablespoons basil, chopped
- 4 tablespoons parmesan, grated
- 1 tablespoon olive oil
- 1 eggplant, cut into medium pieces

Directions:
Grease your Crockpot with the oil, add tomatoes, garlic, onion, salt, pepper, stock, bay leaf, coconut cream, basil and eggplant, cover and cook on Low for 5 hours. Add parmesan, toss, divide between plates and serve as a side dish.
Enjoy!

Nutrition: calories 180, fat 2, fiber 3, carbs 5, protein 10

Creamy Radish Mix

Preparation time: 10 minutes
Cooking time: 3 hours
Servings: 2

Ingredients:

- 14 ounces radishes, halved
- 4 tablespoons coconut cream
- 4 bacon slices, chopped
- 1 tablespoon green onion, chopped
- 1 tablespoon cheddar cheese, grated
- Salt and black pepper to the taste

Directions:
In your Crockpot, mix radishes with cream, bacon, green onion, salt and pepper, toss, cover and cook on High for 3 hours. Divide between plates and serve as a side dish with cheese sprinkled on top.
Enjoy!

Nutrition: calories 340, fat 23, fiber 3, carbs 6, protein 15

Ketogenic Crock Pot Snack And Appetizer Recipes

Simple Cashew Spread

Preparation time: 10 minutes
Cooking time: 6 hours
Servings: 4

Ingredients:
- 5 tablespoons cashews, soaked for 12hours and blended
- 1 teaspoon apple cider vinegar
- 1 cup veggie stock
- 1 tablespoon water

Directions:
In your Crockpot, mix cashews and stock, stir, cover and cook on Low for 6 hours. Drain, transfer to your food processor, add vinegar and water, pulse well, divide between bowls and serve as a party spread.
Enjoy!

Nutrition: calories 221, fat 6, fiber 5, carbs 9, protein 3

Beef Party Rolls

Preparation time: 10 minutes
Cooking time: 8 hours
Servings: 4

Ingredients:
- ½ pounds beef, minced
- 1 green cabbage head, leaves separated
- ½ cup onion, chopped
- 1 cup cauliflower rice
- 2 ounces white mushrooms, chopped
- ¼ cup pine nuts, toasted
- ¼ cup raisins
- 2 garlic cloves, minced
- 2 tablespoons dill, chopped
- 1 tablespoon olive oil
- 25 ounces tomato sauce
- A pinch of salt and black pepper
- ¼ cup water

Directions:
In a bowl, mix beef with onion, cauliflower, mushrooms, pine nuts, raisins, garlic, dill, salt and pepper and stir. Arrange cabbage leaves on a working surface, divide beef mix and wrap them well. Add sauce and water to your Crockpot, stir, add cabbage rolls, cover and cook on Low for 8 hours. Arrange rolls on a platter and serve as an appetizer with some of the sauce from the pot drizzled all over.
Enjoy!

Nutrition: calories 361, fat 6, fiber 6, carbs 12, protein 3

Eggplant And Tomato Salsa

Preparation time: 10 minutes
Cooking time: 7 hours
Servings: 4

Ingredients:
- 1 and ½ cups tomatoes, chopped
- 3 cups eggplant, cubed
- 2 teaspoons capers
- 6 ounces green olives, pitted and sliced
- 4 garlic cloves, minced
- 2 teaspoons balsamic vinegar
- 1 tablespoon basil, chopped
- Salt and black pepper to the taste

Directions:
In your Crockpot, mix tomatoes with eggplant, capers, green olives, garlic, vinegar, basil, salt and pepper, toss, cover and cook on Low for 7 hours. Divide salsa Into small bowls and serve as an appetizer.
Enjoy!

Nutrition: calories 200, fat 6, fiber 5, carbs 9, protein 2

Carrots And Cauliflower Spread

Preparation time: 10 minutes
Cooking time: 7 hours
Servings: 4

Ingredients:
- 1 cup carrots, sliced
- 1 and ½ cups cauliflower florets
- 1/3 cup cashews, soaked for a couple of hours and drained
- ½ cup turnips, chopped
- 2 and ½ cups water
- 1 cup coconut milk
- 1 teaspoon garlic powder
- ¼ cup nutritional yeast
- ¼ teaspoon smoked paprika
- ¼ teaspoon mustard powder
- A pinch of salt and black pepper

Directions:
In your Crockpot, mix carrots with cauliflower, cashews, turnips and water, stir, cover and cook on Low for 7 hours. Drain, transfer to a blender, add milk, garlic powder, yeast, paprika, mustard powder, salt and pepper, blend well, divide between bowls and serve as a party spread.
Enjoy!

Nutrition: calories 291, fat 7, fiber 4, carbs 14, protein 3

Mixed Veggies Spread

Preparation time: 10 minutes
Cooking time: 5 hours
Servings: 7

Ingredients:

- ½ cauliflower head, riced
- 54 ounces canned tomatoes, crushed
- 10 ounces white mushrooms, chopped
- 2 cups carrots, shredded
- 2 cups eggplant, cubed
- 6 garlic cloves, minced
- 2 tablespoons agave nectar
- 2 tablespoons balsamic vinegar
- 2 tablespoons tomato paste
- 1 tablespoon basil, chopped
- 1 and ½ tablespoons oregano, chopped
- 1 and ½ teaspoons rosemary, dried
- A pinch of salt and black pepper

Directions:

In your Crockpot, mix cauliflower with tomatoes, mushrooms, carrots, eggplant, garlic, agave nectar, vinegar, tomato paste, rosemary, salt and pepper, stir, cover and cook on High for 5 hours. Add basil and oregano, stir again, blend a bit using an immersion blender, divide between bowls and serve as a spread.
Enjoy!

Nutrition: calories 301, fat 7, fiber 6, carbs 10, protein 6

Cashew Hummus

Preparation time: 10 minutes
Cooking time: 3 hours
Servings: 4

Ingredients:

- 1 cup water
- 1 cup cashews
- 2 tablespoons tahini paste
- ¼ teaspoon garlic powder
- ¼ teaspoon onion powder
- ¼ cup nutritional yeast
- A pinch of salt and black pepper
- ¼ teaspoon mustard powder
- 1 teaspoon apple cider vinegar

Directions:

In your Crockpot, mix water with cashews, yeast, salt and pepper, stir, cover and cook on High for 3 hours. Transfer to your blender, add tahini, garlic powder, onion powder, mustard powder and vinegar, pulse well, divide between bowls and serve.
Enjoy!

Nutrition: calories 192, fat 7, fiber 7, carbs 12, protein 4

Spinach And Chestnuts Dip

Preparation time: 10 minutes
Cooking time: 1 hour
Servings: 4

Ingredients:
- 1 cup coconut cream
- 10 ounces spinach, torn
- 8 ounces water chestnuts, chopped
- 1 garlic clove, minced
- Black pepper to the taste

Directions:
In your Crockpot, mix coconut cream with spinach, chestnuts, black pepper and garlic, stir, cover and cook on High for 30 minutes. Blend using an immersion blender, divide between bowls and serve as a party dip.
Enjoy!

Nutrition: calories 241, fat 5, fiber 7, carbs 12, protein 5

Bell Peppers Appetizer

Preparation time: 10 minutes
Cooking time: 4 hours and 10 minutes
Servings: 5

Ingredients:
- 1 yellow onion, chopped
- 2 teaspoons olive oil
- 2 celery ribs, chopped
- 1 tablespoon chili powder
- 3 garlic cloves, minced
- 2 teaspoon cumin, ground
- 1 and ½ teaspoon oregano, dried
- 2 and ½ cups cauliflower rice
- 1 tomato chopped
- 1 chipotle pepper In adobo
- A pinch of salt and black pepper
- 5 colored bell peppers, tops and Insides scooped out
- ½ cup tomato sauce

Directions:
Heat up a pan with the oil over medium- high heat, add onion and celery, stir and cook for 5 minutes. Add garlic, chili, cumin, oregano, cauliflower, tomato, chipotle, salt and pepper, stir, cook for a couple of minutes more, take off heat and stuff peppers with this mix. Arrange bell peppers In your Crockpot, spread tomato sauce over them, cover, cook on Low for 4 hours, arrange on a platter and serve them as an appetizer.
Enjoy!

Nutrition: calories 221, fat 5, fiber 4, carbs 9, protein 3

Artichoke And Coconut Spread

Preparation time: 10 minutes
Cooking time: 2 hours
Servings: 8

Ingredients:
- 28 ounces canned artichokes, drained and chopped
- 10 ounces spinach
- 8 ounces coconut cream
- 1 yellow onion, chopped
- 2 garlic cloves, minced
- ¾ cup coconut milk
- ½ cup feta cheese, crumbled
- 1/3 cup mayonnaise
- 1 tablespoon red vinegar
- A pinch of salt and black pepper

Directions:
In your Crockpot, mix artichokes with spinach, coconut cream, onion, garlic, coconut milk, cheese, mayo, vinegar, salt and pepper, stir well, cover and cook on Low for 2 hours. Whisk spread well, divide between bowls and serve as an appetizer.
Enjoy!

Nutrition: calories 305, fat 14, fiber 4, carbs 9, protein 13

Mushroom And Bell Peppers Spread

Preparation time: 10 minutes
Cooking time: 4 hours
Servings: 6

Ingredients:
- 2 cups green bell peppers, chopped
- 1 cup yellow onion, chopped
- 3 garlic cloves, minced
- 1 pound mushrooms, chopped
- 28 ounces tomato sauce
- Salt and black pepper to the taste

Directions:
In your Crockpot, mix bell peppers with onion, garlic, mushrooms, tomato sauce, salt and pepper, stir, cover and cook on Low for 4 hours. Divide between bowls and serve as a spread.
Enjoy!

Nutrition: calories 205, fat 4, fiber 7, carbs 9, protein 3

Chicken Wings Appetizer

Preparation time: 10 minutes
Cooking time: 3 hours
Servings: 6

Ingredients:

- 2 tablespoons garlic, minced
- 2 and ¼ cups pineapple juice
- 3 tablespoons coconut aminos
- 1 tablespoon ginger, minced
- 1 teaspoon olive oil
- A pinch of salt and black pepper
- 3 pounds chicken wings
- A pinch of red pepper flakes, crushed
- 2 tablespoons five spice powder
- Chopped cilantro, for serving

Directions:

Put pineapple juice In your Crockpot, add oil, salt, pepper, aminos, ginger and garlic and whisk well. Add chicken wings, pepper flakes and five spice, toss, cover and cook on High for 3 hours. Arrange chicken wings on a platter, drizzle some of the sauce over them, sprinkle cilantro and serve as an appetizer.
Enjoy!

Nutrition: calories 252, fat 4, fiber 4, carbs 9, protein 20

Cod Sticks

Preparation time: 10 minutes
Cooking time: 2 hours
Servings: 4

Ingredients:

- 2 eggs, whisked
- 1 pound cod fillets, cut into medium strips
- 1 and ½ cups almond flour
- A pinch of salt and black pepper to the taste
- ½ cup tapioca flour
- ¼ teaspoon paprika
- Cooking spray

Directions:

In a bowl, mix almond flour, salt, pepper, tapioca and paprika and stir. Put the eggs In another bowl. Dip fish sticks In the egg, dredge In flour mix, arrange them In your Crockpot after you've greased it with cooking spray, cover and cook on High for2 hours. Arrange cod sticks on a platter and serve.
Enjoy!

Nutrition: calories 261, fat 2, fiber 4, carbs 7, protein 12

Crock Pot Pecans Snack

Preparation time: 10 minutes
Cooking time: 2 hours and 20 minutes
Servings: 5

Ingredients:

- 1 pound pecans, halved
- 2 tablespoons olive oil
- 1 teaspoon basil, dried
- 1 tablespoon chili powder
- 1 teaspoon oregano, dried
- ¼ teaspoon garlic powder
- 1 teaspoon thyme, dried
- ½ teaspoon onion powder

Directions:

In your Crockpot, mix pecans with oil, basil, chili powder, oregano, garlic powder, onion powder and thyme, toss to coat, cover, cook on High for 20 minutes and on Low for 2 hours. Divide between bowls and serve as a snack.
Enjoy!

Nutrition: calories 78, fat 3, fiber 2, carbs 9, protein 2

Party Meatballs

Preparation time: 10 minutes
Cooking time: 4 hours
Servings: 4

Ingredients:

- 1 and ½ pounds beef, ground
- 2 small yellow onions, chopped
- 1 egg
- A pinch of salt and black pepper
- 3 tablespoons cilantro, chopped
- 14 ounces canned coconut milk
- 2 tablespoons hot sauce
- 1 teaspoon basil, dried
- 1 tablespoon green curry paste
- 1 tablespoon coconut aminos

Directions:

Put the meat In a bowl, add onions, egg, salt, pepper and 1 tablespoon cilantro, stir well, shape medium sized meatballs and place them In your Crockpot. Add hot sauce, aminos, coconut milk, curry paste, the rest of the cilantro and basil, toss to cover all meatballs and cook on Low for 4 hours. Arrange meatballs on a platter and serve them as an appetizer.
Enjoy!

Nutrition: calories 260, fat 6, fiber 2, carbs 8, protein 4

Shrimp, Mussels And Clams Appetizer

Preparation time: 10 minutes
Cooking time: 6 hours
Servings: 4

Ingredients:

- 1 pound shrimp, peeled and deveined
- 2 pounds mussels, cleaned and debearded
- 28 ounces canned clams
- 1 yellow onion, chopped
- 10 ounces canned tomato paste

Directions:

In your Crockpot, mix shrimp with mussels, clams, onion and tomato paste, stir, cover and cook on Low for 6 hours. Divide Into small bowls and serve as an appetizer.
Enjoy!

Nutrition: calories 200, fat 3, fiber 2, carbs 7, protein 5

Curried Shrimp Appetizer

Preparation time: 10 minutes
Cooking time: 4 hours and 30 minutes
Servings: 2

Ingredients:

- 1 small yellow onion, chopped
- 1 pound shrimp, deveined and peeled
- 15 baby carrots
- 2 garlic cloves, minced
- 1 small green bell pepper, chopped
- 8 ounces canned coconut milk
- 3 tablespoons tomato paste
- ½ teaspoon red pepper, crushed
- ¾ tablespoons curry powder

Directions:

In your food processor, mix onion with garlic, bell pepper, tomato paste, coconut milk, red pepper and curry powder, blend well, add to your Crockpot, also add baby carrots, cover and cook on Low for 4 hours. Add shrimp, stir and cook on Low for 30 minutes more. Divide between bowls and serve as an appetizer.
Enjoy!

Nutrition: calories 200, fat 4, fiber 3, carbs 4, protein 5

Stuffed Chicken Breast Appetizer

Preparation time: 10 minutes
Cooking time: 6 hours
Servings: 4

Ingredients:

- 4 chicken breasts, skinless and boneless
- 1 tablespoon olive oil
- 1 small yellow onion, chopped
- 2 chili peppers, chopped
- 1 small red bell pepper, chopped
- 2 teaspoons garlic, minced
- 6 ounces spinach
- 1 and ½ teaspoon oregano, chopped
- 1 tablespoon lemon juice
- 1 cup veggie stock
- A pinch of salt and black pepper
- A handful parsley, chopped

Directions:

Heat up a pan with the oil over medium- high heat, add bell pepper, chili peppers and onions, stir and cook for 3 minutes. Add spinach, garlic, salt, pepper and oregano, stir, cook for a couple more seconds and take off heat. Cut a pocket In each chicken breast, stuff with spinach mix, arrange In your Crockpot, add stock over them, cover and cook on Low for 6 hours. Arrange stuffed chicken on a platter, sprinkle parsley on top, drizzle the lemon juice and serve.
Enjoy!

Nutrition: calories 245, fat 4, fiber 3, carbs 8, protein 14

Pecans Snack

Preparation time: 10 minutes
Cooking time: 3 hours
Servings: 4

Ingredients:

- 1 cup coconut sugar
- 1 and ½ tablespoon cinnamon powder
- 1 egg white
- 2 teaspoons vanilla extract
- 4 cups pecans
- ¼ cup water
- Cooking spray

Directions:

In a bowl, mix coconut sugar with cinnamon and stir. In another bowl, mix the egg white with vanilla and whisk well. Grease your Crockpot with cooking spray, add pecans, egg white mix and coconut sugar mix as well, toss, cover and cook on Low for 3 hours. Divide pecans mix Into bowls and serve as a snack.
Enjoy!

Nutrition: calories 172, fat 3, fiber 5, carbs 8, protein 2

Spicy Cauliflower Dip

Preparation time: 10 minutes
Cooking time: 2 hours and 15 minutes
Servings: 6

Ingredients:

- 4 bacon slices, chopped and cooked
- 2 jalapenos, chopped
- ½ cup coconut cream
- 2 cups cauliflower rice
- ¼ cup cheddar cheese, grated
- A pinch of salt and black pepper
- 2 tablespoons chives, chopped

Directions:
In your Crockpot, mix bacon with jalapenos, coconut cream, cauliflower, salt and pepper, stir, cover and cook on Low for 2 hours. Add cashew cheese and chives, cover, cook on Low for 15 minutes more, divide between bowls and serve as a party dip
Enjoy!

Nutrition: calories 242, fat 3, fiber 3, carbs 7, protein 6

Spicy Nuts Mix

Preparation time: 10 minutes
Cooking time: 4 hours
Servings: 20

Ingredients:

- 4 tablespoons coconut oil, melted
- 1 ounce Italian seasoning
- 1 teaspoon cinnamon powder
- Cayenne pepper to the taste
- 2 cups cashews
- 2 cups pecans
- 2 cups almonds
- 2 cups walnuts

Directions:
In your Crockpot, mix oil with Italian seasoning, cinnamon, cayenne, cashews, pecans, almonds and walnuts, toss well, cover, cook on Low for 4 hours, divide between bowls and serve as a party snack.
Enjoy!

Nutrition: calories 200, fat 4, fiber 3, carbs 7, protein 4

Veggie Party Mix

Preparation time: 10 minutes
Cooking time:2 hours
Servings: 8

Ingredients:

- 2 eggplants, cubed
- 3 celery stalks, chopped
- 1 pound plum tomatoes, chopped
- 1 zucchini, halved and sliced
- 1 red bell pepper, chopped
- 1 cup sweet onion, chopped
- 3 tablespoons tomato paste
- ½ cup raisins
- 1 tablespoon stevia
- 1 teaspoon red pepper flakes, crushed
- ¼ cup basil, chopped
- ¼ cup parsley, chopped
- A pinch of salt and black pepper
- ¼ cup green olives, pitted and chopped
- ¼ cup capers
- 2 tablespoons red wine vinegar

Directions:

In your Crockpot, mix the eggplants with celery, tomatoes, zucchini, bell pepper, sweet onion, tomato paste, raisins, stevia, pepper flakes, basil, parsley, salt, pepper, olives, capers and vinegar, stir, cover, cook on High for2 hours, divide between bowls and serve as an appetizer.
Enjoy!

Nutrition: calories 80, fat 1, fiber 2, carbs 6, protein 1

Walnuts And Pumpkin Seeds Snack

Preparation time: 10 minutes
Cooking time:2 hours and 30 minutes
Servings: 12

Ingredients:

- Cooking spray
- 1 cup walnuts, chopped
- 1 cup pumpkin seeds
- 2 tablespoons dill, dried
- 2 tablespoons olive oil
- 1 teaspoon rosemary, dried
- 1 tablespoon lemon peel, grated

Directions:

Grease your Crockpot with cooking spray, add walnuts, pumpkin seeds, oil, dill, rosemary and lemon peel, toss, cover and cook on Low for2 hours and 30 minutes. Divide Into bowls and serve as a snack.
Enjoy!

Nutrition: calories 100, fat 2, fiber 2, carbs 3, protein 2

Coconut Crab Spread

Preparation time: 10 minutes
Cooking time: 2 hours
Servings: 6

Ingredients:

- 4 ounces coconut cream
- 1 pound crab meat
- 1 jalapeno, chopped
- 1 red bell pepper, chopped
- 4 tablespoons lemon juice
- 2 garlic cloves, minced
- ½ teaspoon mustard powder

Directions:
In your Crockpot, mix cream with crab meat, jalapeno, bell pepper, lemon juice, garlic and mustard, stir, cover and cook on High for 2 hours. Blend using your immersion blender, divide between bowls and serve as a spread.
Enjoy!

Nutrition: calories 202, fat 3, fiber 6, carbs 7, protein 3

Tomato And Sweet Onion Dip

Preparation time: 10 minutes
Cooking time: 5 hours
Servings: 12

Ingredients:

- 8 pounds tomatoes, peeled and chopped
- 2 sweet onions, chopped
- 6 garlic cloves, minced
- 6 ounces tomato paste
- ¼ cup white vinegar
- 2 tablespoons coconut sugar
- 1 and ½ tablespoons Italian seasoning
- A pinch of salt and black pepper
- ½ cup basil, chopped
- 1 tablespoon thyme, chopped

Directions:
In your Crockpot, mix tomatoes with onions, garlic, tomato paste, vinegar, coconut sugar, Italian seasoning, salt, pepper, basil and thyme, stir, cover, cook on High for 5 hours, blend using an immersion blender, divide between bowls and serve as a dip.
Enjoy!

Nutrition: calories 182, fat 3, fiber 6, carbs 8, protein 3

Mussels And Veggies Appetizer

Preparation time: 10 minutes
Cooking time: 2 hours
Servings: 4

Ingredients:

- 2 pounds mussels, scrubbed
- 2 tablespoons olive oil
- 1 yellow onion, chopped
- 1 teaspoon parsley, dried
- 1 zucchini, sliced
- 1 carrot, sliced
- ½ teaspoon red pepper flakes, crushed
- 2 teaspoons garlic, minced
- 14 ounces tomatoes, chopped
- ½ cup chicken stock

Directions:
In your Crockpot, mix mussels with oil, onion parsley, pepper flakes, garlic, zucchini, carrots, tomatoes and stock, stir, cover and cook on High for 2 hours. Divide between bowls and serve as an appetizer.
Enjoy!

Nutrition: calories 230, fat 2, fiber 3, carbs 7, protein 2

Cheese Dip

Preparation time: 10 minutes
Cooking time: 2 hours and 30 minutes
Servings: 13

Ingredients:

- 8 ounces cream cheese
- A pinch of salt and black pepper
- 16 ounces coconut cream
- 8 ounces pepper jack cheese, chopped
- 15 ounces canned tomatoes mixed with habaneros
- 1 pound Italian sausage, ground
- ¼ cup green onions, chopped

Directions:
Heat up a pan over medium heat, add sausage, stir, brown for a few minutes and transfer to your Crockpot. Add tomatoes mixed with habaneros, salt, pepper, green onions, pepper jack cheese, cream cheese and coconut cream, cover and cook on High for 2 hours and 30 minutes. Stir your dip really well, divide between bowls and serve.
Enjoy!

Nutrition: calories 184, fat 12, fiber 1, carbs 3, protein 6

Different Cream Cheese Dip

Preparation time: 10 minutes
Cooking time: 2 hours
Servings: 4

Ingredients:

- 4 ounces cream cheese, soft
- ½ cup mozzarella cheese, shredded
- ¼ cup parmesan, grated
- ¼ cup coconut cream
- Salt and black pepper to the taste
- 1/2 cup tomato sauce
- ¼ cup mayonnaise
- 1 tablespoon green bell pepper, chopped
- 6 pepperoni slices, chopped
- ½ teaspoon Italian seasoning
- 4 black olives, pitted and chopped

Directions:
In your Crockpot, mix cream cheese with mozzarella, parmesan, cream, salt, pepper, tomato sauce, mayo, bell pepper, Italian seasoning and pepperoni, cover and cook on High for 2 hours. Divide dip Into bowls, sprinkle olives all over and serve.
Enjoy!

Nutrition: calories 400, fat 14, fiber 4, carbs 4, protein 15

Zucchini And Tomato Dip

Preparation time: 10 minutes
Cooking time: 2 hours
Servings: 4

Ingredients:

- 1 cup mozzarella, shredded
- ¼ cup tomato sauce
- 3 zucchinis, roughly chopped
- Salt and black pepper to the taste
- A pinch of cumin
- Cooking spray

Directions:
Spray your Crockpot with cooking spray, add zucchinis, tomato sauce, salt, pepper and cumin, cover and cook on High for 2 hours. Add mozzarella, stir really well, blend a bit using your immersion blender, divide Into small bowls and serve as a dip.
Enjoy!

Nutrition: calories 140, fat 4, fiber 2, carbs 6, protein 4

Zucchini Hummus

Preparation time: 10 minutes
Cooking time: 2 hours
Servings: 5

Ingredients:

- 4 cups zucchinis, chopped
- 1 cup chicken stock
- ¼ cup olive oil
- Salt and black pepper to the taste
- 4 garlic cloves, minced
- ¾ cup tahini
- ½ cup lemon juice
- 1 tablespoon cumin, ground

Directions:
In your Crockpot, mix zucchinis with stock, salt, pepper and cumin, cover, cook on High for 2 hours and transfer to your blender, Add oil, garlic, lemon juice and tahini, blend really well, divide Into small bowls and serve.
Enjoy!

Nutrition: calories 80, fat 5, fiber 3, carbs 6, protein 7

Beef Jerky Snack

Preparation time: 6 hours
Cooking time: 5 hours
Servings: 6

Ingredients:

- 24 ounces amber
- 2 cups chicken stock
- ½ cup Worcestershire sauce
- 2 tablespoons black peppercorns
- 2 tablespoons black pepper
- 2 pounds beef round, sliced

Directions:
In a bowl, mix soy sauce with black peppercorns, black pepper and Worcestershire sauce and whisk well. Add beef slices, toss to coat, leave aside In the fridge for 6 hours, transfer everything to your Crockpot, cover and cook on Low for 5 hours. Divide between bowls and serve.
Enjoy!

Nutrition: calories 300, fat 12, fiber 4, carbs 10, protein 8

Stuffed Mushrooms

Preparation time: 10 minutes
Cooking time: 4 hours
Servings: 5

Ingredients:

- ¼ cup mayonnaise
- 1 teaspoon garlic powder
- 1 cup chicken stock
- 1 small yellow onion, chopped
- 24 ounces white mushroom caps
- Salt and black pepper to the taste
- 1 teaspoon curry powder
- 4 ounces cream cheese, soft
- ¼ cup coconut cream
- ½ cup Mexican cheese, shredded
- 1 cup shrimp, cooked, peeled, deveined and chopped

Directions:

In a bowl, mix mayo with garlic powder, onion, curry powder, cream cheese, coconut cream, cheese, shrimp, salt and pepper to the taste, whisk well and stuff mushrooms with this mix. Transfer mushrooms to your Crockpot, add the stock over them, cover and cook on Low for 4 hours. Arrange mushrooms on a platter and serve as an appetizer.
Enjoy!

Nutrition: calories 244, fat 20, fiber 3, carbs 7, protein 14

Cheesy Party Wings

Preparation time: 10 minutes
Cooking time: 5 hours
Servings: 6

Ingredients:

- 6 pounds chicken wings, halved
- 3 tablespoons chicken stock
- Salt and black pepper to the taste
- ½ teaspoon Italian seasoning
- 2 tablespoons olive oil
- ½ cup parmesan cheese, grated
- A pinch of red pepper flakes, crushed
- 1 teaspoon garlic powder

Directions:

Grease your Crockpot with the oil, add chicken wings, salt, pepper, Italian seasoning, pepper flakes, garlic powder and stock, cover and cook on Low for 5 hours. Add parmesan, toss, divide chicken wings between plates and serve as an appetizer.
Enjoy!

Nutrition: calories 134, fat 8, fiber 1, carbs 5, protein 14

Chicken Rolls

Preparation time:2 hours
Cooking time:2 hours and 30 minutes
Servings: 12

Ingredients:

- 4 ounces blue cheese, crumbled
- 2 cups chicken, cooked and finely chopped
- Salt and black pepper to the taste
- 2 green onions, chopped
- 2 celery stalks, finely chopped
- 1 cup tomato sauce
- ½ teaspoon erythritol
- 12 egg roll wrappers
- 2 tablespoons olive oil

Directions:

In a bowl, mix chicken meat with blue cheese, salt, pepper, green onions, celery, ½ cup tomato sauce and erythritol, stir well and keep In the fridge for2 hours. Place egg wrappers on a working surface, divide chicken mix on them, roll and seal edges. Transfer chicken rolls to your Crockpot, add the rest of the tomato sauce over them, cover an cook on High for2 hours and 30 minutes. Arrange chicken rolls on a platter and serve as an appetizer.
Enjoy!

Nutrition: calories 220, fat 7, fiber 2, carbs 6, protein 10

Zucchini And Cheese Rolls

Preparation time: 10 minutes
Cooking time: 1 hour
Servings: 24

Ingredients:

- 2 tablespoons olive oil
- 3 zucchinis, thinly sliced
- ½ cup tomato sauce
- 24 basil leaves
- 2 tablespoons mint, chopped
- 1 and 1/3 cup ricotta cheese
- Salt and black pepper to the taste
- ¼ cup basil leaves, whole

Directions:

Brush zucchini slices with half of the olive oil, season with salt and pepper, place them on a working surface and leave aside for now. In a bowl, mix ricotta with chopped basil, mint, salt and pepper and stir well. Spread this over zucchini slices, divide whole basil leaves as well, roll, transfer to your Crockpot, add the rest of the oil and the tomato sauce over them, cover and cook on High for 1 hour. Arrange on a platter and serve as an appetizer.
Enjoy!

Nutrition: calories 100, fat 3, fiber 3, carbs 6, protein 2

Salmon Cakes

Preparation time: 10 minutes
Cooking time: 2 hours
Servings: 4

Ingredients:

- 2 garlic cloves, minced
- 1 yellow onion, chopped
- 1 pound wild salmon, boneless and minced
- ¼ cup chives, chopped
- 1 egg
- 2 tablespoons Dijon mustard
- 1 tablespoon coconut flour
- Salt and black pepper to the taste

For the sauce:

- 4 garlic cloves, minced
- 2 tablespoons olive oil
- 2 tablespoons Dijon mustard
- Juice and zest of 1 lemon
- 2 cups coconut cream
- 2 tablespoons chives, chopped

Directions:

In a bowl, mix onion, 2 garlic cloves, salmon, ¼ cup chives, coconut flour, salt, pepper, 2 tablespoons mustard and egg and stir well. Shape medium cakes and put them In your Crockpot. Add 4 garlic cloves, the oil, 2 tablespoons mustard, lemon zest, lemon juice, coconut cream and chives, cover and cook on High for2 hours. Arrange salmon meatballs on a platter, drizzle some of the cooking sauce over them and serve as an appetizer.
Enjoy!

Nutrition: calories 171, fat 5, fiber 1, carbs 6, protein 16

Salmon Salsa

Preparation time: 30 minutes
Cooking time: 1 hour
Servings: 4

Ingredients:

- 4 salmon fillets, skinless, boneless and cubed
- 1 tablespoon olive oil
- A pinch of salt and black pepper
- 1 teaspoon cumin, ground
- 1 teaspoon sweet paprika
- ½ teaspoon ancho chili powder
- 1 teaspoon onion powder

For the salsa:

- 1 small red onion, chopped
- 1 avocado, pitted, peeled and chopped
- 2 tablespoons cilantro, chopped
- Juice of 2 limes
- Salt and black pepper to the taste

Directions:

In a bowl, mix salt, pepper, chili powder, onion powder, paprika and cumin. Rub salmon with this mix, drizzle the oil and transfer to your Crockpot. Add onion, cilantro, lime juice, salt and pepper, toss a bit, cover and cook on High for 1 hour. Divide Into small bowls and serve as an appetizer with avocado sprinkled on top.
Enjoy!

Nutrition: calories 300, fat 14, fiber 4, carbs 5, protein 20

Tuna Cakes

Preparation time: 10 minutes
Cooking time: 1 hour and 20 minutes
Servings: 12

Ingredients:

- 15 ounces canned tuna, drained and flaked
- 3 eggs
- ½ teaspoon dill, dried
- 1 teaspoon parsley, dried
- ½ cup red onion, chopped
- 1 teaspoon garlic powder
- Salt and black pepper to the taste
- ½ cup tomato sauce
- A drizzle of olive oil

Directions:
In a bowl, mix tuna with salt, pepper, dill, parsley, onion, garlic powder and eggs, stir well, shape your cakes, transfer to your Crockpot after you've greased it with some oil, add tomato sauce, cover and cook on High for 1 hour and 20 minutes. Arrange on a platter and serve as an appetizer.
Enjoy!

Nutrition: calories 140, fat 2, fiber 1, carbs 6, protein 6

Creole Shrimp Appetizer

Preparation time: 10 minutes
Cooking time: 1 hour
Servings: 2

Ingredients:

- ½ pound big shrimp, peeled and deveined
- 2 teaspoons Worcestershire sauce
- 2 teaspoons olive oil
- 1 cup chicken stock
- Juice of 1 lemon
- Salt and black pepper to the taste
- 1 teaspoon Creole seasoning

Directions:
Grease your Crockpot with oil, add shrimp, Worcestershire sauce, stock, lemon juice, salt, pepper and Creole seasoning, cover and cook on High for 1 hour. Arrange shrimp on a platter and serve.
Enjoy!

Nutrition: calories 120, fat 3, fiber 1, carbs 2, protein 6

Octopus Salad

Preparation time: 10 minutes
Cooking time: 5 hours
Servings: 2

Ingredients:
- 21 ounces octopus, rinsed
- Juice of 1 lemon
- 4 celery stalks, chopped
-
- 3 ounces olive oil
- Salt and black pepper to the taste
- 4 tablespoons parsley, chopped

Directions:
Put the octopus your Crockpot, add water to cover, salt and pepper, cover and cook on Low for 5 hours. Drain octopus, chop, put In a salad bowl, add lemon juice, celery, oil, salt, pepper and parsley, toss and serve as an appetizer.
Enjoy!

Nutrition: calories 140, fat 10, fiber 3, carbs 6, protein 13

Cod Appetizer Salad

Preparation time:2 hours and 10 minutes
Cooking time: 3 hours
Servings: 8

Ingredients:
- 2 cups jarred pimiento peppers, chopped
- 2 pounds salt cod
- 1 cup parsley, chopped
- 1 cup kalamata olives, pitted and chopped
- 6 tablespoons capers
- ¾ cup olive oil
- Salt and black pepper to the taste
- Juice of 2 lemons
- 4 garlic cloves, minced
- 2 celery ribs, chopped
- ½ teaspoon red chili flakes
- 1 lettuce head, leaves separated

Directions:
Put cod In your Crockpot, add water to cover, cook on Low for 3 hours, drain and transfer to a salad bowl. Add pimiento peppers, parsley, olives, capers, celery, garlic, lemon juice, salt, pepper, olive oil and chili flakes and toss to coat. Arrange lettuce leaves on a platter, add the cod salad and serve.
Enjoy!

Nutrition: calories 240, fat 4, fiber 2, carbs 6, protein 9

Hot Salmon Bites

Preparation time: 10 minutes
Cooking time: 2 hours and 10 minutes
Servings: 6

Ingredients:

- 1 and ¼ cups coconut, desiccated and unsweetened
- 1 pound salmon, cubed
- 1 egg
- Salt and black pepper
- 1 tablespoon water
- 1/3 cup coconut flour
- 3 tablespoons coconut oil

For the sauce:

- ¼ teaspoon agar agar
- 3 garlic cloves, chopped
- ¾ cup water
- 4 Thai red chilies, chopped
- ¼ cup balsamic vinegar
- ½ cup stevia
- A pinch of salt

Directions:
In a bowl, mix flour with salt and pepper and stir. In another bowl, whisk egg and 1 tablespoon water. Put the coconut In a third bowl. Dip salmon cubes In flour, egg and then In coconut and place them on a plate. Heat up a pan with the coconut oil over medium- high heat, add salmon bites, cook for 3 minutes on each side and transfer them to a plate. In your Crockpot, mix ¾ cup water with red chilies, garlic, agar agar, vinegar, stevia and salt, stir, add salmon bites, cover and cook on High for 2 hours. Arrange salmon biter on a platter and serve.
Enjoy!

Nutrition: calories 100, fat 2, fiber 4, carbs 7, protein 12

Salmon Salad

Preparation time: 10 minutes
Cooking time: 1 hour
Servings: 2

Ingredients:

- 2 medium salmon fillets
- ½ cup seafood stock
- Salt and black pepper to the taste
- A drizzle of olive oil
- 1 shallot, chopped
- 1 lettuce head, leaves torn
- 1 tablespoon lemon juice
- ¼ cup olive oil
- 2 tablespoons parsley, finely chopped

Directions:
Brush salmon fillets with a drizzle of olive oil, sprinkle with salt and pepper, put them In your Crockpot, add stock, cover and cook on High for 1 hour. Meanwhile, put shallot In a bowl, add 1 tablespoon lemon juice, salt and pepper, stir and leave aside for 10 minutes. Flake salmon, put In a bowl, add lettuce leaves, shallot, the rest of the oil and parsley, toss and serve as an appetizer.
Enjoy!

Nutrition: calories 200, fat 10, fiber 1, carbs 5, protein 16

Chili Dip

Preparation time: 10 minutes
Cooking time: 2 hours
Servings: 8

Ingredients:

- 5 ancho chilies, dried and chopped
- 2 garlic cloves, minced
- Slat and black pepper to the taste
- 1 and ½ cups water
- 2 tablespoons balsamic vinegar
- 1 and ½ teaspoons stevia
- 1 tablespoon oregano, chopped
- ½ teaspoon cumin, ground

Directions:
In your Crockpot mix water chilies, garlic, salt, pepper, stevia, cumin and oregano, stir, cover and cook on High for 2 hours. Blend using an immersion blender, add vinegar, stir, divide between bowls and serve as a snack.
Enjoy!

Nutrition: calories 85, fat 1, fiber 1, carbs 2, protein 2

Beets Dip

Preparation time: 10 minutes
Cooking time: 3 hours
Servings: 8

Ingredients:

- 1 yellow onion, chopped
- 2 tablespoons olive oil
- 5 celery ribs
- 8 garlic cloves, minced
- 8 carrots, chopped
- 4 beets, peeled and chopped
- 1 butternut squash, peeled and chopped
- 1 cup veggie stock
- ¼ cup lemon juice
- 1 bunch basil, chopped
- 2 bay leaves
- Salt and black pepper to the taste

Directions:
Grease your Crockpot with the oil, add celery, carrots, onions, beets, squash, garlic, stock, lemon juice, basil, bay leaves, salt and pepper, stir, cover and cook on High for 3 hours. Discard bay leaves, blend using an immersion blender, divide between bowls and serve.
Enjoy!

Nutrition: calories 143, fat 1, fiber 3, carbs 4, protein 3

Mango Dip

Preparation time: 10 minutes
Cooking time: 1 hour and 20 minutes
Servings: 4

Ingredients:
- 1 shallot, chopped
- 1 tablespoon coconut oil
- ¼ teaspoon cardamom powder
- 2 tablespoons ginger, minced
- ½ teaspoon cinnamon powder
- 2 mangos, peeled and chopped
- 2 red hot chilies, chopped
- 1 apple, cored and chopped
- ¼ cup raisins
- 5 tablespoons stevia
- 1 and ¼ tablespoon balsamic vinegar

Directions:
Grease your Crockpot with the oil, shallot, ginger, cinnamon, hot peppers, cardamom, mangos, apple, raisins, stevia and vinegar, stir, cover and cook on High for 1 hour and 20 minutes
Transfer to bowls and serve cold.
Enjoy!

Nutrition: calories 100, fat 2, fiber 1, carbs 3, protein 1

Balsamic Mushrooms Dip

Preparation time: 10 minutes
Cooking time: 2 hours
Servings: 4

Ingredients:
- 6 ounces mushrooms, chopped
- 3 tablespoon olive oil
- 1 tablespoon thyme, chopped
- 1 garlic clove, minced
- 4 ounces beef stock
- 1 tablespoon balsamic vinegar
- 1 tablespoon mustard
- 2 tablespoon coconut cream
- 2 tablespoons parsley, finely chopped

Directions:
Grease your Crockpot with the oil, add thyme, mushrooms, garlic, vinegar, stock, mustard, coconut cream and parsley, stir, cover and cook on High for 2 hours. Stir really well, divide between bowls and serve as a snack.
Enjoy!

Nutrition: calories 140, fat 3, fiber 2, carbs 4, protein 3

Clams And Mussels Appetizer Salad

Preparation time: 10 minutes
Cooking time: 2 hours
Servings: 4

Ingredients:

- 15 small clams
- 30 mussels, scrubbed
- 2 chorizo links, sliced
- 1 yellow onion, chopped
- 10 ounces veggie stock
- 2 tablespoons parsley, chopped
- 1 teaspoon olive oil
- Lemon wedges for serving

Directions:
Grease your Crockpot with the oil and add onion and chorizo on the bottom. Add clams, mussels, stock and parsley, toss, cover and cook on High for 2 hours. Divide Into small bowls and serve with lemon wedges on the side.
Enjoy!

Nutrition: calories 172, fat 4, fiber 3, carbs 7, protein 12

Easy Clams Delight

Preparation time: 10 minutes
Cooking time: 1 hour and 20 minutes
Servings: 4

Ingredients:

- 24 clams, shucked
- 3 garlic cloves, minced
- 2 tablespoons coconut oil
- ¼ cup parsley, chopped
- ¼ cup parmesan cheese, grated
- 1 teaspoon oregano, dried
- 1 cup almonds, crushed
- 1 and ½ cups seafood stock
- Lemon wedges

Directions:
In a bowl, mix almonds with parmesan, oregano, parsley, coconut oil and garlic, stir and divide this Into exposed clams. Add the stock to your Crockpot, add clams Inside, cover and cook on High 1 hour and 20 minutes. Arrange clams on a platter and serve them as an appetizer with lemon wedges on the side.
Enjoy!

Nutrition: calories 92, fat 3, fiber 3, carbs 6, protein 5

Artichokes Appetizer

Preparation time: 10 minutes
Cooking time: 2 hours
Servings: 4

Ingredients:

- 4 big artichokes, trimmed
- Salt and black pepper to the taste
- 2 tablespoons lemon juice
- ¼ cup olive oil
- 2 teaspoons balsamic vinegar
- 1 teaspoon oregano, dried
- 2 garlic cloves, minced
- 1 cup chicken stock

Directions:
In your Crockpot, mix stock with oil, vinegar, oregano, garlic, lemon juice, salt and pepper and whisk. Add artichokes, toss a bit, cover and cook on High for 2 hours. Arrange artichokes on a platter and serve as an appetizer.
Enjoy!

Nutrition: calories 162, fat 4, fiber 2, carbs 3, protein 5

Endives Appetizer Salad

Preparation time: 10 minutes
Cooking time: 3 hours
Servings: 4

Ingredients:

- 4 endives, trimmed
- 1 cup chicken stock
- Salt and black pepper to the taste
- 2 tablespoons coconut oil
- 4 slices ham, roughly chopped
- ½ teaspoon nutmeg, ground
- 14 ounces coconut cream

Directions:
In your Crockpot, mix endives with stock, salt, pepper, oil, ham, nutmeg and coconut cream, cover and cook on High for 3 hours. Divide Into small bowls and serve as an appetizer.
Enjoy!

Nutrition: calories 152, fat 3, fiber 3, carbs 6, protein 12

Ketogenic Crock Pot Dessert Recipes

Cocoa Pudding

Preparation time: 10 minutes
Cooking time: 1 hour
Servings: 2

Ingredients:

- 2 tablespoons water
- 2 tablespoon gelatin
- 4 tablespoons stevia
- 4 tablespoons cocoa powder
- 2 cups coconut milk, hot

Directions:

In a bowl, mix milk with stevia and cocoa powder and stir well. In a bowl, mix gelatin with water, stir well, add to the cocoa mix, stir and transfer to your Crockpot. Cover, cook on High for 1 hours, divide between bowls and keep In the fridge until you serve it.
Enjoy!

Nutrition: calories 120, fat 2, fiber 1, carbs 4, protein 3

Raspberry Bars

Preparation time: 10 minutes
Cooking time: 1 hour
Servings: 12

Ingredients:

- ½ cup coconut butter
- ½ cup coconut oil
- ½ cup coconut, unsweetened and shredded
- 1 cup raspberries
- 3 tablespoons coconut sugar

Directions:

In your Crockpot, mix coconut butter with coconut oil, coconut, raspberries and sugar, toss, cover and cook on High for 1 hour. Spread on a lined baking sheet, keep In the fridge for a few hours, slice and serve.
Enjoy!

Nutrition: calories 174, fat 5, fiber 2, carbs 4, protein 7

Mascarpone And Berries Cream

Preparation time: 10 minutes
Cooking time: 1 hour
Servings: 12

Ingredients:

- 8 ounces mascarpone cheese
- ¾ teaspoon coconut sugar
- 1 cup coconut cream
- ½ pint blueberries
- ½ pint strawberries

Directions:

In your Crockpot, mix cream with stevia, mascarpone, blueberries and strawberries, stir, cover and cook on Low for 1 hour. Divide Into small dessert bowls and serve cold.
Enjoy!

Nutrition: calories 183, fat 4, fiber 1, carbs 3, protein 1

Simple Orange Cake

Preparation time: 10 minutes
Cooking time: 4 hours
Servings: 12

Ingredients:

- 6 eggs
- 1 orange, peeled and cut into quarters
- 1 teaspoon vanilla extract
- Cooking spray
- 1 teaspoon baking powder
- 9 ounces almond meal
- 4 tablespoons coconut sugar
- 2 tablespoons orange zest, grated
- 2 ounces stevia
- 4 ounces cream cheese
- 4 ounces coconut cream

Directions:

In your food processor, mix orange with almond meal, sugar, eggs, baking powder and vanilla extract, pulse well and transfer to your Crockpot after you've greased it with cooking spray and lined with parchment paper. Cook on High for 4 hours and transfer cake to a cake plate. In a bowl, mix cream cheese with orange zest, coconut cream and stevia and stir well. Spread this well over cake, slice and serve it.
Enjoy!

Nutrition: calories 170, fat 13, fiber 2, carbs 4, protein 4

Berry Pudding

Preparation time: 10 minutes
Cooking time: 1 hour
Servings: 4

Ingredients:
- 3 tablespoons cocoa powder
- 14 ounces coconut cream
- 1 cup blackberries
- 1 cup raspberries
- 2 tablespoons stevia

Directions:
In your Crockpot, mix cream with cocoa, stevia, blackberries and raspberries, stir, cover and cook on High for 1 hour. Divide Into dessert cups and serve cold.
Enjoy!

Nutrition: calories 145, fat 4, fiber 2, carbs 6, protein 2

Stewed Peaches

Preparation time: 10 minutes
Cooking time: 1 hour and 30 minutes
Servings: 6

Ingredients:
- 4 tablespoons coconut sugar
- 3 cups peaches, cored and roughly chopped
- 6 tablespoons natural apple juice
- 2 teaspoons lemon zest, grated

Directions:
In your Crockpot, mix peaches with sugar, apple juice and lemon zest, stir, cover and cook at High for 1 hour and 30 minutes. Divide Into small cups and serve cold.
Enjoy!

Nutrition: calories 100, fat 2, fiber 2, carbs 5, protein 5

Almond And Cocoa Cake

Preparation time: 10 minutes
Cooking time: 4 hours
Servings: 4

Ingredients:
- ½ teaspoon almond extract
- 1 cup coconut flour
- ½ cup cocoa powder
- Cooking spray
- 4 tablespoons coconut sugar
- 3 tablespoons olive oil
- 3 eggs
- 2 teaspoons baking powder
- ½ cup almonds, sliced

Directions:
In a bowl, mix cocoa powder, almond extract, flour, eggs, coconut sugar, oil, baking powder and almonds, whisk well and pour everything Into your Crockpot after you've greased it with cooking spray. Cover, cook on High for 4 hours, leave aside to cool down, slice, divide between plates and serve.
Enjoy!

Nutrition: calories 202, fat 4, fiber 2, carbs 8, protein 3

Pumpkin And Cauliflower Pudding

Preparation time: 30 minutes
Cooking time: 3 hours
Servings: 6

Ingredients:
- 1 cup cauliflower rice
- ½ cup water
- 3 cups coconut milk
- ½ cup dates, chopped
- 1 teaspoon cinnamon powder
- 1 cup pumpkin puree
- 4 tablespoons coconut sugar
- 1 teaspoon vanilla extract

Directions:
Put cauliflower rice In your Crockpot, add water, milk, dates, coconut sugar, vanilla, pumpkin and cinnamon, stir, cover and cook on High for 3 hours. Divide pudding Into bowls and serve.
Enjoy!

Nutrition: calories 120, fat 3, fiber 3, carbs 8, protein 5

Berries Marmalade

Preparation time: 10 minutes
Cooking time: 2 hours and 30 minutes
Servings: 8

Ingredients:

- 1 pound cranberries
- 1 pound strawberries
- ½ pound blueberries
- 3.5 ounces black currant
- Coconut sugar to the taste
- Zest of 1 lemon, grated
- ½ cup water

Directions:

In your Crockpot, mix strawberries with cranberries, blueberries, currants, lemon zest, coconut sugar and water, stir, cover and cook on High for 2 hours and 30 minutes. Divide Into dessert cups and serve cold.
Enjoy!

Nutrition: calories 100, fat 0, fiber 1, carbs 7, protein 3

Zucchini Cake

Preparation time: 10 minutes
Cooking time: 4 hours
Servings: 6

Ingredients:

- 1 cup natural applesauce
- 3 eggs, whisked
- 1 tablespoon vanilla extract
- 4 tablespoons coconut sugar
- 2 cups zucchini, grated
- 2 and ½ cups coconut flour
- ½ cup baking cocoa powder
- 1 teaspoon baking soda
- ¼ teaspoon baking powder
- 1 teaspoon cinnamon powder
- ½ cup walnuts, chopped
- Cooking spray

Directions:

Grease your Crockpot with cooking spray, add zucchini, sugar, vanilla, eggs, applesauce, flour, cocoa powder, baking soda, baking powder, cinnamon and walnuts, whisk well, cover and cook on High for 4 hours. Leave the cake to cool down, slice and serve.
Enjoy!

Nutrition: calories 192, fat 3, fiber 6, carbs 8, protein 3

Carrots Dessert

Preparation time: 10 minutes
Cooking time: 1 hour
Servings: 4

Ingredients:
- 1 tablespoon stevia
- 2 cups baby carrots
- 1 tablespoon ghee, melted
- ½ cup water

Directions:
In your Crockpot, mix carrots with stevia, ghee and water, stir, cover and cook on High for 1 hour. Divide Into dessert cups and serve them cold.
Enjoy!

Nutrition: calories 120, fat 1, fiber 1, carbs 2, protein 2

Pear Pudding

Preparation time: 5 minutes
Cooking time: 1 hour
Servings: 4

Ingredients:
- 2 cups pears, chopped
- 2 cups coconut milk
- 1 tablespoon ghee, melted
- 3 tablespoons stevia
- ½ teaspoon cinnamon powder
- 1 cup coconut flakes
- ½ cup walnuts, chopped

Directions:
In your Crockpot, mix milk with stevia, ghee, coconut, cinnamon, pears and walnuts, stir, cover and cook on High for 1 hour. Divide between bowls and serve cold.
Enjoy!

Nutrition: calories 172, fat 3, fiber 4, carbs 8, protein 7

Coconut Bars

Preparation time: 10 minutes
Cooking time: 1 hour
Servings: 10

Ingredients:
- ½ cup coconut butter
- ½ cup coconut oil
- ½ cup raspberries, dried
- ¼ cup coconut sugar
- ½ cup coconut, shredded

Directions:
In your food processor, blend dried berries very well, transfer to your Crockpot, add coconut butter, coconut oil, sugar and coconut, stir really well, cover and cook on High for 1 hour. Transfer to a lined baking sheet, keep In the fridge for a few hours, slice and serve.
Enjoy!

Nutrition: calories 234, fat 12, fiber 2, carbs 4, protein 2

Berries And Cream Dessert

Preparation time: 10 minutes
Cooking time: 1 hour
Servings: 4

Ingredients:
- 3 tablespoons cocoa powder
- 14 ounces coconut cream
- 1 cup blackberries
- 1 cup raspberries
- 2 tablespoons stevia

Directions:
In your Crockpot, whisk cocoa powder with stevia, cream, blackberries and raspberries, cover, cook on High for 1 hour, divide Into dessert cups and serve cold.
Enjoy!

Nutrition: calories 205, fat 34, fiber 2, carbs 6, protein 2

Almonds And Coconut Granola

Preparation time: 10 minutes
Cooking time: 3 hours
Servings: 4

Ingredients:

- 1 cup coconut, unsweetened and shredded
- 1 cup almonds, chopped
- 2 tablespoons coconut sugar
- ½ cup pumpkin seeds
- ½ cup sunflower seeds
- 3 tablespoons coconut oil
- 1 teaspoon nutmeg, ground
- 1 teaspoon apple pie spice mix

Directions:
In a bowl, mix almonds with pumpkin seeds, sunflower seeds, coconut, nutmeg and apple pie spice mix and stir well. Grease your Crockpot with the oil, add sugar and almond mix, whisk, spread well Into the pot, cover and cook on High for 3 hours. Transfer the mix to a lined baking sheet, spread well, leave aside to cool down, slice and serve.
Enjoy!

Nutrition: calories 120, fat 2, fiber 2, carbs 4, protein 5

Cherry Marmalade

Preparation time: 10 minutes
Cooking time: 3 hours
Servings: 6

Ingredients:

- 2 tablespoons lemon juice
- 3 tablespoons gelatin
- 4 cups cherries, pitted
- 2 cups coconut sugar

Directions:
In your Crockpot, mix lemon juice with gelatin, cherries and coconut sugar, stir, cover and cook on High for 3 hours. Divide Into cups and serve cold.
Enjoy!

Nutrition: calories 211, fat 3, fiber 1, carbs 3, protein 3

Simple Cauliflower Pudding

Preparation time: 10 minutes
Cooking time: 5 hours
Servings: 4

Ingredients:
- 2 and ½ cups water
- 1 cup coconut sugar
- 2 cups cauliflower rice
- 2 cinnamon sticks
- ½ cup coconut, shredded

Directions:
In your Crockpot, mix water with coconut sugar, cauliflower rice, cinnamon and coconut, stir, cover and cook on High for 5 hours. Divide pudding Into cups and serve cold.
Enjoy!

Nutrition: calories 113, fat 4, fiber 6, carbs 9, protein 4

Pumpkin Cake

Preparation time: 10 minutes
Cooking time: 2 hours and 20 minutes
Servings: 10

Ingredients:
- 1 and ½ teaspoons baking powder
- Cooking spray
- 1 cup pumpkin puree
- 2 cups almond flour
- ½ teaspoon baking soda
- 1 and ½ teaspoons cinnamon powder
- ¼ teaspoon ginger, ground
- 1 tablespoon coconut oil, melted
- 1 tablespoon flax meal
- 1 tablespoon vanilla extract
- 1/3 cup maple syrup
- 1 teaspoon lemon juice

Directions:
In a bowl, flour with baking powder, baking soda, cinnamon, ginger, flaxseed, oil, vanilla, pumpkin puree, maple syrup and lemon juice and whisk well. Grease your Crockpot with cooking spray, pour cake mix, cover and cook on Low for 2 hours and 20 minutes. Leave the cake to cool down, slice and serve.
Enjoy!

Nutrition: calories 182, fat 3, fiber 2, carbs 3, protein 1

Strawberries And Blueberries Marmalade

Preparation time: 10 minutes
Cooking time: 4 hours
Servings: 10

Ingredients:
- 14 ounces strawberries, chopped
- 20 ounces blueberries
- 2 pounds coconut sugar
- Zest of1 lemon, grated
- 4 ounces raisins
- 3 ounces water

Directions:
In your Crockpot, mix strawberries with coconut sugar, lemon zest, raisins and water, stir, cover and cook on High for 4 hours. Divide Into small jars and serve cold.
Enjoy!

Nutrition: calories 100, fat 3, fiber 2, carbs 2, protein 1

Lemon Marmalade

Preparation time: 10 minutes
Cooking time: 3 hours
Servings: 10

Ingredients:
- 2 pounds lemons, washed, peeled and sliced
- 2 pounds coconut sugar
- 1 tablespoon white vinegar

Directions:
In your Crockpot, mix lemons with coconut sugar and vinegar, stir, cover and cook on High for 3 hours. Divide Into jars and serve cold.
Enjoy!

Nutrition: calories 100, fat 0, fiber 2, carbs 7, protein 4

Apples Jam

Preparation time: 10 minutes
Cooking time: 5 hours
Servings: 12

Ingredients:
- 2 pounds apples, washed, peeled and sliced
- 2 pounds coconut sugar
- 1 tablespoon cinnamon powder

Directions:
In your Crockpot, mix apples with sugar and cinnamon, stir, cover and cook on Low for 5 hours. Divide between bowls and serve cold.
Enjoy!

Nutrition: calories 100, fat 0, fiber 2, carbs 7, protein 4

Rhubarb And Berries Marmalade

Preparation time: 10 minutes
Cooking time: 3 hours
Servings: 8

Ingredients:
- 1/3 cup water
- 2 pounds rhubarb, chopped
- 2 pounds blueberries, chopped
- 1 cup coconut sugar
- 1 tablespoon mint, chopped

Directions:
In your Crockpot, mix water with rhubarb, berries, sugar and mint, stir, cover and cook on High for 3 hours. Divide Into cups and serve cold.
Enjoy!

Nutrition: calories 100, fat 1, fiber 4, carbs 10, protein 2

Sweet Plums

Preparation time: 10 minutes
Cooking time: 3 hours
Servings: 6

Ingredients:
- 14 plums, pitted and halved
- 1 and ¼ cups palm sugar
- 1 teaspoon cinnamon powder
- ¼ cup water

Directions:
In your Crockpot, mix plums with sugar, cinnamon and water, stir, cover, cook on Low for 3 hours, divide Into cups and serve cold.
Enjoy!

Nutrition: calories 150, fat 2, fiber 1, carbs 2, protein 3

Fruit Bowls

Preparation time: 10 minutes
Cooking time: 2 hours
Servings: 10

Ingredients:
- 3 pears, cored and chopped
- ½ cup raisins
- 2 cups dried fruits
- 1 teaspoon ginger powder
- ¼ cup palm sugar
- 1 teaspoon lemon juice
- 1 teaspoon lemon zest, grated

Directions:
In your Crockpot, mix pears with raisins, dried fruits, ginger, sugar, lemon juice and lemon zest, stir, cover, cook on High for2 hours, divide between bowls and serve cold.
Enjoy!

Nutrition: calories 140, fat 3, fiber 4, carbs 6, protein 6

Sweet Strawberry Cream

Preparation time: 10 minutes
Cooking time: 3 hours
Servings: 10

Ingredients:

- 2 tablespoons lemon juice
- 2 pounds strawberries, chopped
- 4 cups coconut sugar
- 1 teaspoon cinnamon powder
- 1 teaspoon vanilla extract

Directions:
In your Crockpot, mix strawberries with coconut sugar, lemon juice, cinnamon and vanilla, cover and cook on Low for 3 hours. Blend a bit using your immersion blender, divide between bowls and keep In the fridge until you serve it.
Enjoy!

Nutrition: calories 100, fat 0, fiber 1, carbs 2, protein 2

Apple Stew

Preparation time: 10 minutes
Cooking time: 4 hours
Servings: 6

Ingredients:

- 6 apples, cored, peeled and sliced
- 1 and ½ cups almond flour
- Cooking spray
- 1 cup coconut sugar
- 1 tablespoon cinnamon powder
- ¾ cup cashew butter, melted

Directions:
Grease your Crockpot with cooking spray, add apples, flour, sugar, cinnamon and coconut butter, stir gently, cover, cook on High for 4 hours, divide between bowls and serve cold.
Enjoy!

Nutrition: calories 180, fat 5, fiber 5, carbs 8, protein 4

Berry Pie

Preparation time: 10 minutes
Cooking time: 2 hours
Servings: 6

Ingredients:

- 1 pound fresh blackberries
- 1 pound fresh blueberries
- ¾ cup water
- ¾ cup coconut sugar
- 1 cup tapioca flour
- ½ cup arrowroot powder
- 1 teaspoon baking powder
- 2 tablespoons palm sugar
- 1/3 cup coconut milk
- 1 egg, whisked
- 1 teaspoon lemon zest, grated
- 3 tablespoons coconut oil, melted

Directions:
In your Crockpot, mix blueberries, blackberries, coconut sugar, water and half of the tapioca, cover and cook on High for 1 hour. Meanwhile, In a bowl, mix the rest of the tapioca flour with arrowroot with palm sugar and baking powder and stir well. Add egg, milk, oil and lemon zest, stir, drop spoonfuls of this mix over the berries from the Crockpot, cover and cook on High for 1 more hour. Leave pie aside to cool down, divide Into dessert bowls and serve.
Enjoy!

Nutrition: calories 240, fat 4, fiber 3, carbs 6, protein 6

Simple Orange Pudding

Preparation time: 10 minutes
Cooking time: 5 hours
Servings: 4

Ingredients:

- Cooking spray
- 1 teaspoon baking powder
- 1 cup almond flour
- 1 cup palm sugar
- ½ teaspoon cinnamon, ground
- 3 tablespoons coconut oil, melted
- ½ cup almond milk
- ½ cup pecans, chopped
- ¾ cup water
- ½ cup raisins
- ½ cup orange peel, grated
- ¾ cup orange juice

Directions:
In a bowl, mix flour with half of the sugar, baking powder and cinnamon and stir. Add 2 tablespoons oil, milk, pecans and raisins, stir and pour this Into Crockpot after you've greased it with cooking spray. Heat up a small pan over medium- high heat, add water, orange juice, orange peel, the rest of the oil and the rest of the sugar, stir, bring to a simmer, pour over the mix In the Crockpot, cover and cook on Low for 5 hours. Divide Into dessert bowls and serve.
Enjoy!

Nutrition: calories 182, fat 3, fiber 1, carbs 8, protein 6

Stuffed Apples

Preparation time: 10 minutes
Cooking time:2 hours
Servings: 4

Ingredients:

- 4 apples, tops cut off and cored
- 4 figs
- 4 tablespoons coconut sugar
- 1 teaspoon ginger powder
- ¼ cup pecans, chopped
- 2 teaspoons lemon zest, grated
- ¼ teaspoon nutmeg, ground
- ½ teaspoon cinnamon powder
- 1 tablespoon lemon juice
- 1tablespoon coconut oil
- ½ cup water

Directions:
In a bowl, mix figs with sugar, ginger, pecans, lemon zest, nutmeg, cinnamon, oil and lemon juice, whisk really well and stuff your apples with this mix. Put the water In your Crockpot, arrange apples, cover, cook on High for2 hours, divide on dessert plates and serve.
Enjoy!

Nutrition: calories 200, fat 1, fiber 2, carbs 4, protein 7

Chocolate Cake

Preparation time: 10 minutes
Cooking time: 3 hours
Servings: 10

Ingredients:

- 1 cup almond flour
- ½ cup cocoa powder
- ½ cup coconut sugar
- 1 and ½ teaspoons baking powder
- 3 eggs
- Cooking spray
- 4 tablespoons coconut oil, melted
- ¾ teaspoon vanilla extract
- 2/3 cup almond milk
- 1/3 cup dark chocolate chips

Directions:
In a bowl, mix swerve with almond flour, cocoa powder, baking powder, milk, oil, eggs, chocolate chips and vanilla extract, whisk really well, pour this Into your lined and greased Crockpot and cook on Low for 3 hours. Leave the cake aside to cool down, slice and serve.
Enjoy!

Nutrition: calories 200, fat 12, fiber 4, carbs 8, protein 6

Stewed Pears

Preparation time: 10 minutes
Cooking time: 4 hours
Servings: 4

Ingredients:

- 4 pears, peeled and tops cut off and cored
- 5 cardamom pods
- 2 cups apple juice
- ¼ cup maple syrup
- 1 cinnamon stick
- 1 Inch ginger, grated

Directions:
Put the pears In your Crockpot, add cardamom pods, apple juice, maple syrup, cinnamon and ginger, cover and cook on Low for 4 hours. Divide between bowls and serve with the sauce drizzled on top.
Enjoy!

Nutrition: calories 200, fat 4, fiber 2, carbs 3, protein 4

Maple Pecans

Preparation time: 10 minutes
Cooking time: 1 hour
Servings: 3

Ingredients:

- 2 teaspoons vanilla extract
- 3 cups pecans
- ¼ cup maple syrup
- 1 tablespoon coconut oil

Directions:
Put your pecans In the Crockpot, add vanilla extract, oil and maple syrup, toss to coat and cook on High for 1 hour. Divide Into cups and serve.
Enjoy!

Nutrition: calories 200, fat 2, fiber 2, carbs 4, protein 7

Plum And Cinnamon Compote

Preparation time: 10 minutes
Cooking time:2 hours
Servings: 10

Ingredients:

- 4 pounds plums, stones removed and cut into medium wedges
- 1 cup water
- 2 tablespoons palm sugar
- 1 teaspoon cinnamon powder

Directions:
Put plums, water, sugar and cinnamon In your Crockpot, cover and cook on Low for2 hours. Divide bowls and serve cold.
Enjoy!

Nutrition: calories 103, fat 0, fiber 1, carbs 2, protein 4

Passion Fruit Dessert Cream

Preparation time: 10 minutes
Cooking time: 4 hours
Servings: 6

Ingredients:

- 1 cup passion fruit juice
- 4 passion fruits, pulp and seeds separated
- 3 and ½ ounces maple syrup
- 3 eggs
- 2 ounces coconut oil, melted
- 3 and ½ ounces coconut milk
- ½ cup almond flour
- ½ teaspoon baking powder

Directions:
In your Crockpot, mix juice with passion fruits pulp and seeds, maple syrup, eggs, coconut, almond milk, almond flour and baking powder, whisk really well, cover and cook on Low for 4 hours. Whisk really well, divide between bowls and serve cold.
Enjoy!

Nutrition: calories 230, fat 12, fiber 3, carbs 7, protein 8

Cherry And Cocoa Compote

Preparation time: 10 minutes
Cooking time: 4 hours
Servings: 6

Ingredients:

- ½ cup dark cocoa powder
- ¾ cup cherry juice
- ¼ cup maple syrup
- 1 pound cherries, pitted and halved
- 2 tablespoons stevia
- 2 cups water

Directions:
In your Crockpot, mix cocoa powder with cherry juice, maple syrup, cherries, water and stevia, stir, cover and cook on Low for 4 hours. Divide between bowls and serve cold.
Enjoy!

Nutrition: calories 207, fat 1, fiber 4, carbs 5, protein 2

Grapefruit And Mint Compote

Preparation time: 10 minutes
Cooking time: 4 hours
Servings: 6

Ingredients:

- 1 cup water
- 1 cup maple syrup
- ½ cup mint, chopped
- 64 ounces red grapefruit juice
- 2 grapefruits, peeled and chopped

Directions:
In your Crockpot, mix grapefruit with water, maple syrup, mint and grapefruit juice, stir, cover and cook on Low for 4 hours. Divide between bowls and serve cold.
Enjoy!

Nutrition: calories 120, fat 1, fiber, 2, carbs 2, protein 1

Maple Figs Stew

Preparation time: 10 minutes
Cooking time: 1 hour
Servings: 4

Ingredients:

- 2 tablespoons coconut butter
- 12 figs, halved
- 1 cup almonds, chopped
- ¼ cup maple syrup

Directions:
In your Crockpot, mix coconut butter with maple syrup, whisk well, add figs and almonds, toss, cover and cook on Low for 1 hour. Divide between bowls and serve right away.
Enjoy!

Nutrition: calories 170, fat 6, fiber 5, carbs 6, protein 8

Special Apple Cake

Preparation time: 10 minutes
Cooking time:2 hours and 30 minutes
Servings: 6

Ingredients:

- 3 cups apples, cored and cubed
- 1 cup coconut sugar
- 1 tablespoon vanilla
- 2 eggs
- 1 tablespoon pumpkin pie spice
- 2 cups almond flour
- 1 tablespoon baking powder
- 1 tablespoon ghee, melted

Directions:
In your Crockpot, mix apples with coconut sugar, vanilla, eggs, apple pie spice, almond flour, baking powder and ghee, cover and cook on High for2 hours and 20 minutes. Leave the special cake to cool down, slice and serve.
Enjoy!

Nutrition: calories 170, fat 2, fiber 4, carbs 12, protein 4

Vanilla Espresso Cream

Preparation time: 10 minutes
Cooking time: 1 hour and 30 minutes
Servings: 4

Ingredients:
- 1 cup coconut milk
- 1 cup hemp hearts
- 2 and ½ cups water
- 2 tablespoons coconut sugar
- 1 teaspoon espresso powder
- 2 teaspoons vanilla extract

Directions:
In your Crockpot, mix hemp with water, sugar, milk and espresso powder, stir, cover and cook on High for 1 hour and 30 minutes Add vanilla extract, stir, divide between bowls and serve cold Enjoy!

Nutrition: calories 200, fat 4, fiber 6, carbs 12, protein 4

Lemon And Blackberries Cream

Preparation time: 30 minutes
Cooking time: 1 hour
Servings: 4

Ingredients:
- 1 cup coconut milk
- Zest of1 lemon, grated
- 6 egg yolks
- 1 cup coconut cream
- 1 cup water
- 2/3 cup coconut sugar
- ½ cup fresh blackberries

Directions:
In your Crockpot, mix coconut milk with lemon zest, whisked egg yolks, cream, water, coconut sugar and blackberries, toss, cover and cook on High for 1 hour. Divide between bowls and serve cold.
Enjoy!

Nutrition: calories 162, fat 4, fiber 6, carbs 9, protein 4

Stewed Figs

Preparation time: 10 minutes
Cooking time: 1 hour and 20 minutes
Servings: 4

Ingredients:
- 1 cup red grape juice
- 1 pound figs
- ½ cup pine nuts, toasted
- ½ cup coconut sugar

Directions:
In your Crockpot, mix figs with grape juice, coconut sugar and pine nuts, toss, cover and cook on High for 1 hour and 20 minutes. Divide stewed figs Into small bowls and serve them cold. Enjoy!

Nutrition: calories 132, fat 4, fiber 3, carbs 7, protein 4

Carrot Cake

Preparation time: 10 minutes
Cooking time: 4 hours
Servings: 4

Ingredients:
- 5 ounces almond flour
- ¾ teaspoon baking powder
- ½ teaspoon baking soda
- ½ teaspoon cinnamon powder
- ¼ teaspoon nutmeg, ground
- ½ teaspoon allspice
- 1 egg
- 3 tablespoons coconut cream
- ½ cup coconut sugar
- ¼ cup pineapple juice
- 4 tablespoons coconut oil, melted
- ½ cup carrots, grated
- 1/3 cup pecans, toasted and chopped
- 1/3 cup coconut flakes
- Cooking spray

Directions:
In a bowl, mix flour with baking soda and powder, allspice, cinnamon and nutmeg and stir. In a second bowl, mix the egg with coconut cream, sugar, pineapple juice, oil, carrots, pecans and coconut flakes and stir well. Combine the two mixtures, stir very well everything, pour this Into your Crockpot after you've greased it with cooking spray, cover and cook on Low for 4 hours. Leave the cake to cool down, then cut and serve it. Enjoy!

Nutrition: calories 251, fat 4, fiber 4, carbs 7, protein 4

Peach Marmalade

Preparation time: 10 minutes
Cooking time: 3 hours
Servings: 6

Ingredients:
- 4 and ½ cups peaches, peeled and cubed
- 6 cups coconut sugar
- 2 tablespoons ginger, grated
- ½ cup water

Directions:
In your Crockpot, mix peaches with sugar, ginger and water, stir, cover and cook on High for 3 hours. Divide marmalade Into jars and serve as a dessert.
Enjoy!

Nutrition: calories 100, fat 0, fiber 3, carbs 6, protein 4

Raspberry Cream

Preparation time: 10 minutes
Cooking time: 2 hours
Servings: 4

Ingredients:
- 1 cup coconut sugar
- 12 ounces raspberries
- 2 egg yolks, whisked
- 2 tablespoons lemon juice
- 2 tablespoons coconut oil, melted

Directions:
In your Crockpot, mix raspberries with sugar, egg yolks, lemon juice and melted coconut oil, whisk well, cover and cook on High for 2 hours. Whisk your cream one more time, divide Into small cups and serve cold.
Enjoy!

Nutrition: calories 123, fat 4, fiber 4, carbs 7, protein 3

Dried Fruits Pudding

Preparation time: 10 minutes
Cooking time: 3 hours
Servings: 4

Ingredients:

- 4 ounces dried cranberries, soaked In hot water, drained and chopped
- A drizzle of avocado oil
- 4 ounces dried apricots, chopped
- 1 cup almond flour
- 3 teaspoons baking powder
- 1 cup coconut sugar
- 1 teaspoon ginger powder
- ½ teaspoon cinnamon powder
- 15 tablespoons ghee, melted
- 3 tablespoons maple syrup
- 4 eggs
- 1 carrot, grated

Directions:

In a blender, mix flour with baking powder, sugar, cinnamon, salt and ginger and pulse a few times. Add ghee, maple syrup, eggs, dried cranberries, dried apricots and carrot, fold them Into the batter and spread this Into your Crockpot after you've greased it with a drizzle of avocado oil. Cover, cook on Low for 3 hours, leave aside to cool down, divide between bowls and serve. Enjoy!

Nutrition: calories 271, fat 4, fiber 6, carbs 12, protein 4

Peach Cake

Preparation time: 10 minutes
Cooking time: 4 hours
Servings: 6

Ingredients:

- 1/8 teaspoon almond extract
- 1 cup peaches, pitted and chopped
- 4 tablespoons coconut flour
- ½ cup cocoa powder
- ½ cup coconut sugar
-
- 3 tablespoons avocado oil
- 3 eggs
- 2 teaspoons baking powder
- ¼ cup almonds, sliced

Directions:

In a bowl, mix almond extract with peaches, flour, cocoa, sugar, oil, eggs, baking powder and almonds, whisk well, transfer to your Crockpot after you've greased it with cooking spray, cover and cook on Low for 4 hours. Leave the cake to cool down, slice and serve. Enjoy!

Nutrition: calories 164, fat 4, fiber 6, carbs 8, protein 4

Ricotta And Dates Cake

Preparation time: 30 minutes
Cooking time: 4 hours
Servings: 6

Ingredients:
- 1 pound ricotta
- 6 oz dates, soaked for 15 minutes and drained
- 3 ounces coconut sugar
- 4 eggs
- ½ teaspoon vanilla extract
- Zest of ½ lemon, grated
- Cooking spray

Directions:
In a bowl, whisk ricotta until it softens. Add eggs, sugar, dates, vanilla and lemon zest, whisk well, pour Into your Crockpot after you've greased it with cooking spray, cover and cook on Low for 4 hours. Leave the cake to cool down, slice and serve.
Enjoy!

Nutrition: calories 200, fat 6, fiber 6, carbs 8, protein 10

Rhubarb Compote

Preparation time: 10 minutes
Cooking time: 3 hours
Servings: 4

Ingredients:
- 1 cup water
- 2 pounds rhubarb, chopped
- 4 tablespoon coconut sugar
- 1/3 pound strawberries, chopped

Directions:
Put rhubarb, water, sugar and strawberries In your Crockpot, cover and cook on High for 3 hours. Divide between bowls and serve cold.
Enjoy!

Nutrition: calories 100, fat 4, fiber 5, carbs 6, protein 1

Carrot Pudding

Preparation time: 10 minutes
Cooking time: 4 hours
Servings: 8

Ingredients:
- Cooking spray
- ½ cup coconut sugar
- 3 eggs
- ½ cup almond flour
- ½ teaspoon allspice, ground
- ½ teaspoon cinnamon powder
- A pinch of nutmeg
- ½ teaspoon baking soda
- 2/3 cup ghee, melted
- ½ cup pecans, chopped
- 1 cup carrots, grated
- ½ cup raisins

Directions:
In a bowl, mix sugar with eggs, almond flour, allspice, cinnamon, nutmeg, baking soda, melted ghee, pecans, carrots and raisins, stir well, pour Into your Crockpot after you've greased it with cooking spray, cover and cook on Low for 4 hours. Leave carrot pudding to cool down, slice and serve.
Enjoy!

Nutrition: calories 200, fat 4, fiber 6, carbs 12, protein 4

Chestnut Cream

Preparation time: 10 minutes
Cooking time: 3 hours
Servings: 6

Ingredients:
- 11 ounces coconut sugar
- 11 ounces water
- 1 and ½ pounds chestnuts, halved and peeled

Directions:
In your Crockpot, mix sugar with water and chestnuts, stir, cover and cook on Low for 3 hours. Blend using your immersion blender, divide Into small cups and serve.
Enjoy!

Nutrition: calories 102, fat 1, fiber 0, carbs 5, protein 3

Conclusion

A Ketogenic diet might be exactly what you need In your life right now! This diet is easy to follow and it brings you so many health benefits!
On the other hand, Crockpots are some of the most popular kitchen appliances available on the market these days.
These wonderful tools help you cook delicious and healthy meals for all your loved ones.

Now, we ask you: what do you get from combining one of the healthiest diets with the best cooking tool?
Well, the answer is pretty simple: you get the cooking experience of a lifetime!
So, don't hesitate! Get your hands on this amazing cooking journal and start your new and improved life!
Start cooking Ketogenic style with your amazing Crockpot!
Enjoy!

Recipe Index

Made in the USA
Lexington, KY
27 March 2018